THE HEALING HIERARCHY

FREE WORKBOOK

Here's what you'll find inside The Healing Hierarchy Implementation Workbook:

- ☑ **The Stability Score Self-Assessment:** Your baseline number, dated, so you can track your progress from start to finish and measure real change
- ☑ **The Timeline That Explains What Happened:** Map the stressors, infections, and events that accumulated before your health declined and pinpoint when things shifted
- ☑ **The "Where Do I Start?" Scoring Exercise:** Score yourself at each of the four levels to find where your recovery should actually begin
- ☑ **Your Foundations Check**: Blood sugar, sleep, movement, and nervous system scored individually so you know which one needs attention first
- ☑ **The Testing Strategy Planner:** Know exactly which tests to request, what clinical question each one answers, and the order to run them
- ☑ **Your System Maps:** Gut, energy, hormones, and mood each scored and mapped so you can see what is actually driving your symptoms
- ☑ **The Decision Tree:** Your score points to one of three clear pathways so you stop guessing and start in the right place

Scan This QR Code below or visit:
TheHealingHierarchy.com/workbook

Get The Workbook
SCAN HERE

The Healing Hierarchy

Restore Function. Rebuild Your Body.

Jarrod Cooper ND

Hierarchy Press

Medical & Health Disclaimer

This book is for informational and educational purposes only. It is not a substitute for professional medical advice, diagnosis, or treatment. Always consult with a qualified healthcare provider before making changes to your health routine, starting new supplements, adopting new dietary practices, or beginning any wellness programme.

The author holds a Bachelor of Health Science (Naturopathy) and is a member of the Australian Natural Therapies Association (ANTA). The information in this book is based on clinical experience, published research, and professional opinion. Individual health outcomes vary significantly based on genetics, medical history, lifestyle, concurrent conditions, and numerous other factors. Nothing in this book constitutes a guarantee of specific results.

The case studies in this book are drawn from real clinical practice. Names, identifying details, and certain clinical specifics have been changed to protect patient privacy. The data and outcomes described are documented but may not be representative of typical results.

The supplement protocols, testing strategies, and dietary recommendations discussed in this book are presented as a clinical framework, not as prescriptions. Do not begin, discontinue, or modify any supplement, medication, or treatment protocol without the guidance of a qualified practitioner familiar with your individual case.

The author and publisher are not liable for any adverse health effects or negative outcomes resulting from the use of or reliance on the information in this book.

ISBN numbers :

Ebook: 978-1-7645711-2-8

Paperback: 978-1-7645711-0-4

Hardback: 978-1-7645711-1-1

Audiobook: 978-1-7645711-3-5

Edition: First Edition

Format: Paperback, Hardback, Ebook and Audiobook

Praise for The Healing Hierarchy

"In The Healing Hierarchy, Dr. Cooper offers a refreshingly clear and practical framework for those who feel like they're doing everything "right," yet still struggling with persistent symptoms. Rather than offering another rigid protocol, this book provides a thoughtful roadmap that helps readers understand what to stabilize first and where to go from there. This is an essential guide for both patients and practitioners seeking a more strategic, sustainable path to true healing."

– Dr. Izabella Wentz, PharmD, The Thyroid Pharmacist, New York Times Bestselling Author of Hashimoto's Protocol

For everyone who has been told nothing is wrong

while everything feels like it is

Acknowledgements

This book exists because thousands of patients trusted me with their health when the conventional system had run out of answers. Every case shaped this framework, every data set refined the sequence, and you are the evidence base this book stands on.

To Gemma, who believed in this work before there was a book, a clinic, or a framework, when it was just an idea and a lot of late nights. She was the one who helped me see that I couldn't do everything at once. That stepping back from clinic time to focus on our family and this book wasn't giving something up, but making room for what mattered most. On the days I wanted to stop, she would not let me. On the days I couldn't see the point, she could. This book exists because of her belief, her patience, and the thousands of small things she did to keep everything moving.

And to every reader holding this book: you aren't broken. You are unmeasured. This book is the map. The rest is yours.

Contents

Introduction

There is a kind of exhaustion that doesn't come from doing too little.

It comes from doing everything right, and watching nothing change.

You didn't ignore your health. If anything, you gave it more attention than most people would ever consider reasonable. You cleaned up the diet. You ran the tests. You took the supplements. You followed the protocols. And yet something shifted — gradually, until the effort you were putting in no longer matched the results you were getting back.

That mismatch, between effort and outcome, is destabilising in a way few people talk about or even consciously recognise.

Because when effort fails, the first place the mind looks is inward. *Maybe I missed something. Maybe I need to try harder. Maybe I need to be stricter.* So you add more. Another protocol. Another supplement. Another layer of restriction. For a while, something improves. Then it doesn't. The improvement fades, or a new symptom appears. Over time, something more subtle begins to erode.

Trust.

Not just trust in practitioners. Trust in your own body.

And that may be the worst part. Not the symptoms themselves, but the slow realisation that the person you have always been – capable, resourceful, someone who solves problems – cannot solve this one. Not for lack of trying. For lack of a framework that matches what your body is doing.

After more than a decade in clinical practice and thousands of complex chronic cases, I can tell you that this pattern is not rare. In fact, it is the most common presentation I see. People who are doing the right things, reliably, and not getting the results those things should produce.

And what struck me most was never how sick these people were. It was how hard they were trying. And how little their effort was being rewarded.

The issue was not lack of information. It was not lack of discipline or commitment. It was lack of structure. People were treating pieces of a system without understanding the system itself. They were stacking inputs without knowing whether their body could process them. Chasing markers without restoring stability. Suppressing signals without asking what generated them.

The turning point in my own practice came when I stopped asking *what protocol matches this diagnosis?* and started asking *why did this system lose its ability to regulate?*

That shift changed outcomes. Once I saw it, I couldn't unsee it.

This book exists because the people who need this understanding most will likely never walk into my clinic. They live in different cities, different countries, different healthcare systems. Some have no access to functional medicine at all. Some have access but are not being guided in the right sequence. Some are doing everything correctly, just in the wrong order.

By the time you finish this book, you will understand why your good days stopped being repeatable, and what that means. You will know what needs to settle before anything else can build. You will stop stacking random interventions and start making decisions in sequence. You will understand how to restore your body's responsiveness before attempting to optimise its performance.

Your body hasn't failed you. It has crossed a threshold, and no one explained what that meant or what to do about it.

This book is that explanation. This book comes with a free companion workbook

— 19 exercises that turn what you read into what you do.

Download yours at TheHealingHierarchy.com/workbook

How to Use This Book

This is not a book you need to rush through. It is, however, a book that works best read in order.

Each chapter builds on the one before it.

The first three chapters establish why your body may have stopped responding and introduce the framework that explains the sequence of recovery.

Chapters 4 through 7 cover the foundations: food, sleep, movement, and nervous system regulation, which must be at least partially in place before the clinical chapters will make full sense.

Chapters 8 and 9 introduce the testing strategy.

Chapters 10 through 13 walk through the major body systems one by one, each anchored by a real patient case.

Chapters 14 through 17 cover protocols, genetics, detoxification, and environmental factors.

Chapter 18 addresses longevity.

Chapter 19 brings the framework together.

If you want one chapter to read first, read Chapter 3 — The Healing Hierarchy. It is the single concept that changes how you evaluate every protocol, practitioner, and supplement you encounter from this point forward.

The Companion Workbook

A free Implementation Workbook is available at TheHealingHierarchy.com/workbook. It includes exercises for every chapter — self-assessments, tracking tools, and reflection prompts designed to take 10–15 minutes each. You don't need the workbook to benefit from this book, but readers who use it report that the exercises make the framework personal rather than theoretical.

The Stability Score

In Chapter 2, you will assess your Stability Score. A zero-to-ten measure of how predictable and resilient your body is right now. This number appears throughout the book as a reference point. Write it down. Date it. You will reassess it in Chapter 19, and the movement in that number will tell you more than any single lab result.

A Note on Case Studies

Every case study in this book is drawn from real clinical practice. Names and identifying details have been changed, but the data is real and the outcomes are documented. These cases are included not as proof that every reader will experience the same result, but as demonstrations of how the framework operates when applied in sequence with the right data.

Estimated Reading Time

The full book takes approximately five to six hours to read cover to cover. But this isn't a book you will read once. Most readers return to specific chapters as they move through their own testing and recovery. Keep it within reach.

PART I

THE TRAP

Chapter One

Doing Everything Right... And Still Not Getting Better

She doesn't look like someone who is unwell.

That is the first thing you notice.

She is composed, articulate, the kind of woman who walks into a room already running through her agenda. She manages a team. She runs a household. She has the sharp focus that belongs to people who have learned to get things done regardless of how they feel.

By every visible measure, she is on top of it.

She sits down, places her phone face-down on the desk — deliberate, and slides over a manila folder.

Inside are blood results from three different practitioners, annotated in her own handwriting. Four months of sleep data, the 2 a.m. wake-ups marked more often than not. A supplement list — sixteen items. Some with question marks beside them. Not doubting the products. Doubting whether they are doing anything at all. Stool tests. Hormone panels. An organic acids report. A GP letter that reads: within normal limits. Consider stress management.

She has done the work.

Gluten removed. Then dairy. Then sugar. Then seed oils. Low-FODMAP. Autoimmune protocol. Ketogenic cycles. An elimination programme so restrictive that dinner became a clinical exercise.

Her supplement cabinet resembles a dispensary. Magnesium. Omega-3. Zinc. Probiotics. Methylation support. Adaptogens. Mitochondrial blends. Half-used bottles from protocols that worked briefly and then stopped.

She walks daily, strength trains carefully, and goes to bed at the same time every night. No alcohol. Tracks heart rate variability and understands what it means.

She has seen specialists. Spent thousands. Read the books. Listened to the podcasts. She knows her ferritin, her TSH, her oestradiol. She can explain reverse T3.

She has discipline. She has data. She has effort — applied consistently for years.

She looks up and says:

"I'm doing everything right. And I'm getting worse, not better."

Not angry. Just tired. And beneath the tiredness, something more corrosive — the erosion of trust. Not just in practitioners. In her own body.

I see this person every week.

Different name. Different folder. Same pattern.

High effort. Low return.

When Effort Stops Working

When effort produces results, failure is useful. You try something, it doesn't work, you adjust, you try again. The feedback loop stays intact.

Even failure feels productive because it narrows the options and moves you closer.

But when effort stops producing results entirely, the feedback loop breaks. You do everything correctly, and nothing moves. The same actions that once created progress now land in silence. You remove another food group, add another supplement, try another practitioner, and the needle does not shift. Or it shifts briefly, just long enough to reignite hope, and then slides back to exactly where it was.

The internal dialogue shifts. First: *what should I try next?* Then, after enough failed attempts: *what am I missing?* Then, quietly, at 3 a.m., staring at the ceiling after another night of fragmented sleep: *is this just how it's going to be now?*

That question is where the real damage begins. Not because the answer is yes. But because asking it means something fundamental has shifted. You are no longer troubleshooting a problem. You are starting to accept a verdict. Acceptance, when it arrives prematurely, does not bring peace. It brings resignation. The kind that sits beneath a perfectly functional exterior and slowly drains the colour out of everything.

From that place, most people do what has always worked for them in every other area of life. They double down. More restriction. More supplements. More testing. More effort. More discipline. Because discipline has always been the answer before.

Sometimes there is a brief lift: energy improves, digestion settles, skin clears, and hope returns. Then it slips again. Or a new symptom appears in place of the old one. The gut calms but the brain fog thickens. The fatigue lifts but the anxiety arrives. The weight shifts but the sleep fragments.

The effort that used to scale no longer does.

And nobody can explain why.

The Cost Nobody Talks About

The cost of this cycle is not just physical. It is the quiet erosion of identity.

These are not people who struggle with discipline. They are people who have built entire lives on competence. They run businesses, lead teams, and manage households with precision. They solve complex problems as a matter of routine, but they can't decode their own body. That gap, between who they are in every other domain and how they feel physically, becomes its own source of shame.

It shows up in ways they rarely talk about. Sitting across from their spouse at dinner, knowing they are only half present. Watching friends eat freely at a restaurant, order without anxiety, travel without planning around symptoms, and feeling an envy that is difficult to admit out loud. Pushing through the afternoon crash with caffeine and sheer will, delivering what the day demands, then collapsing the moment they walk through the door. Cancelling plans. Missing weekends with their children. Turning down opportunities because they don't trust their energy to hold.

They would give up half of what they have earned to feel normal for a week. They have thought that exact sentence, even if they have never said it.

And they won't talk about it. Not to their spouse. Not their doctor. Not their closest friend. Because admitting it means admitting that the thing they have built their identity on, the ability to handle whatever comes, is no longer working.

No one sees it. That is the point.

They are high-functioning. And they are hostage to a body that has stopped cooperating.

The Pattern Behind the Frustration

When someone walks in with that folder: the labs, the supplement list, the failed protocols, the look of controlled exhaustion. I am not looking at a person who has failed.

I am looking at someone whose body has changed the rules without telling them.

There is a particular pattern that shows up across these cases, regardless of the diagnosis on the referral letter. The person is doing the right things, genuinely and consistently. Yet their body isn't responding the way it should.

Sleep should be restorative; it isn't. The diet should be producing stability; it doesn't. The long list of supplements should be building something. Some may be the right call, supporting various metabolic pathways, but many in the extensive protocol are either doing nothing or making things worse. Recovery from exercise, from stress, from a late night, from a challenging meal — all of it takes longer than it should. And the unpredictability may be the hardest part. A good day appears, and for a moment, hope returns. Then it vanishes, without clear explanation, and the crash feels worse than it would have if the good day had never come at all.

This is not a collection of unrelated symptoms. It is a pattern.

And once you see it, you see it everywhere. In the woman with autoimmune disease who cannot tolerate the very supplements designed to help her. In the executive with persistent fatigue whose testosterone is low, but whose fatigue started long before the hormone shifted. In the mother whose body never recovered after pregnancy, not because pregnancy damaged her, but because it was the final demand on a system that was already running without margin. In the athlete who overtrained into a wall and cannot climb back, no matter how much rest and recovery they add.

Different people. Different histories. Different diagnoses.

The same pattern underneath.

The Question Nobody Asked

The woman sitting across from me had seen five practitioners before she walked into my clinic. She had been given diagnoses. She had been given protocols. She had been told her labs were normal, her thyroid was fine, her gut was "probably just IBS." She had been told to manage her stress.

None of them were wrong, exactly. But none of them had asked the question that mattered.

They had asked: *What is the symptom? What do we treat?*

Nobody had asked: *What state is this body in? Does that state explain why nothing is working?*

That is a different question. And it leads to a completely different answer.

Because the same symptom means something completely different depending on the state of the body producing it. Fatigue in a regulated body is a signal — something specific is depleted or disrupted, and correcting it resolves the problem. Fatigue in a body that has lost its ability to regulate is not a single signal. It is the sound of a system that can no longer process its own inputs. Correcting one thing does not resolve it, because the issue is not one thing. The issue is the condition the body is in.

And when the body can't absorb the intervention, the strategy fails. No matter how right the tools are.

That distinction, between treating a symptom and understanding the overall state of the body, is the single most important shift presented in this entire book.

At the end of that first session, she closed the folder. Not in defeat. Not in relief. With something more specific than either. The stillness that settles when three years of confusion finally has a coherent explanation.

She did not leave with a new protocol. She left with a different understanding: her body hadn't stopped working. Something had changed the rules of what the body could tolerate, and that shift had a name.

Chapter Two

Why Your Body Stopped Responding

Your body didn't randomly stop cooperating.

It didn't wake up one morning and decide to ignore everything you were doing for it. It didn't become lazy. It didn't lose interest in healing. Something changed — something structural, something measurable, something that explains why the same inputs that once produced results now produce nothing, or worse.

Once you understand what shifted, the confusion that has been following you for months or years begins to resolve. The answer is not simple, but it is specific.

The Body Is a Network

The human body is not a collection of parts put together to make a whole. It is a network, an organization. The gut communicates with the immune system. The immune system signals the brain. The brain regulates hormones. Hormones influence metabolism. Metabolism fuels every cell. Energy production, detoxification, inflammation control, hormone balance, blood sugar regulation, immune discrimination — these are coordinated processes, each one dependent on the behaviour of the others.

When this network is intact, the body is adaptable. You sleep and wake feeling restored. You eat and energy remains steady. You train and recover.

You handle stress and return to baseline. You get sick and bounce back. The system absorbs variation and recalibrates. Inputs produce predictable outputs.

That predictability is invisible when it is working. You don't notice that your body is coordinating thousands of regulatory conversations every second, because the coordination is seamless. You just feel normal. You feel like yourself.

But that adaptability has a threshold. When the threshold is exceeded, the rules change.

Your Body's Buffer

Think of the threshold as a buffer — your body's ability to absorb stress, process inputs, and return to stability. When the buffer is high, you have margin. You can miss a night of sleep and recover the next day. You can eat something you normally avoid and tolerate it without consequence. You can push through a stressful week and feel tired, but not broken. You can get a virus and fight it off. The system bends without breaking.

When the buffer is low, that margin disappears. Sleep becomes fragile — you wake at 2 a.m. and cannot return to sleep until 5 a.m., only to be woken an hour later exhausted. Foods you tolerated for years begin producing reactions. Stress does not pass through you anymore; it accumulates. Recovery from exercise, from illness, from a long day, takes longer than it should. Symptoms appear, not dramatically at first, but persistently. And the unpredictability becomes its own burden, because you can no longer trust how your body will respond to any given day.

Nothing may look dramatically wrong on paper — your labs may read normal, your scans may be clear. But you can feel your ability to tolerate life shrinking. And you are right.

The buffer is not a metaphor. It is biological. It reflects the combined resilience of your gut integrity, your detoxification pathways, your mitochondrial output, your nervous system regulation, your immune tolerance, and your hormonal signalling. When those systems are functioning, the buffer absorbs the daily demands of living. When they are compromised, even partially, even quietly, the buffer declines. Once it declines far enough, something fundamental changes.

I call that change the Sensitization Threshold.

The Sensitization Threshold

It is the point at which cumulative load exceeds what your body can tolerate. The tipping point where normal inputs begin producing abnormal outputs. The research community calls a related concept *allostatic load*. The cumulative wear on the body's regulatory systems when they are forced to adapt to sustained stress.

Bruce McEwen's work at Rockefeller University established the framework: the body adapts until it can't, and the cost of that adaptation accumulates silently until the system tips. What I see in clinical practice is the human version of that tipping point — the moment the patient notices.

Before this threshold is crossed, the body is forgiving. It compensates. It absorbs stress and recalibrates. After it is crossed, the same inputs produce different outputs.

Fatigue persists despite adequate sleep, weight plateaus despite careful restriction, and gut symptoms continue despite elimination diets. Inflammation remains elevated despite supplementation.

Hormones stay chaotic despite targeted intervention. Good days appear and then vanish without explanation. The body hasn't become lazy. It has become sensitised. Your systems are no longer stable. They are reactive. Small inputs trigger exaggerated responses. The system is operating without a buffer.

From the outside, it looks like a collection of unrelated problems arriving at the same time. From the inside, it is one thing: the body stopped responding predictably.

There is a way to measure where you sit right now. I developed a tool I call the Stability Score. A zero-to-ten self-assessment that tracks not just how you feel on any given day, but how predictable and resilient your body has become over time.

A score of zero to three means crisis: symptoms are unpredictable, recovery from any stressor is slow and disproportionate, and life is organised around managing the illness. Four to six means improving but fragile: good days are appearing, but setbacks are common and the fear of regression is constant. Seven to eight means stable: occasional flares still occur, but they are tied to identifiable triggers and the body recovers within a reasonable timeframe. Nine to ten means resilient: the body handles the demands of daily life without collapsing.

Most people reading this book will recognise themselves somewhere between two and five. And as startling as that may seem, it is not a verdict. It is a starting position. And the purpose of everything that follows: the framework, the testing, the sequenced restoration, is to move that number upward in a way that holds.

You will see the Stability Score referenced throughout this book. It is the single measure that tracks your progress from where you are now to where the framework can take you.

Score Yourself Now

Answer each question honestly based on the last thirty days. Score each 0 (not at all), 1 (sometimes), or 2 (consistently).

1. Can you predict how you will feel tomorrow based on how you feel today?

2. Does your body recover from a poor night's sleep within one day?

3. Can you eat a varied whole-food diet without unexpected reactions?

4. Does your energy hold steady from morning through afternoon without crashing?

5. Can you handle a stressful day without your symptoms flaring for days afterward?

Your total: ______ / 10

0–3: Crisis — your system is sensitised and unpredictable. Start with the foundations in Chapters 3 through 7.

4–6: Improving but fragile — good days are appearing but setbacks are common. The framework in this book will show you why, and what to address next.

7–8: Stable — your body is responding. Focus on optimising and monitoring.

9 10: Resilient — maintain what you have built and watch for drift.

Whatever your score, testing is how you turn this number into a plan. Write your number down. Date it. You will come back to it.

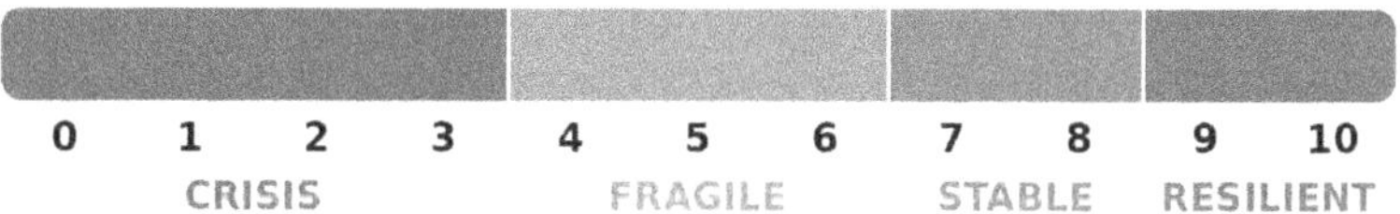

For the full assessment, with personalised recommendations based on your answers, visit TheHealingHierarchy.com/workbook

What Pushes Someone Across

Rarely one thing. Almost always, cumulative load. Even when patients can point to a single event, an infection, a pregnancy, a mold exposure, that event was the final stressor on a system already running out of margin.

Consider a woman in her early forties. She had always been healthy — active, lean, sharp. She ran a business, trained three times a week, ate well. Then she caught a virus that lingered longer than it should have. She pushed through it because that is what she does. Two months later, she was still tired. Then perimenopause arrived, and sleep started fracturing. She was managing — barely, when the renovation at her office introduced mold she did not know about for six months. By the time she sat in front of a practitioner, she had four separate diagnoses and not one of them explained why she had been fine eighteen months ago and was now reacting to everything.

She had not developed four conditions. She had crossed one threshold, and each stressor on its own was manageable. Stacked together, over time, they exceeded what her system could handle.

The specifics vary. For some, it was a virus they never fully recovered from — glandular fever in their twenties, or COVID that left a residue the immune system couldn't clear. For others, it was prolonged stress that was managed but never resolved: years at full capacity while sleeping five hours a night. For some, it was hormonal. A pregnancy that demanded more than the body had in reserve, or perimenopause arriving on top of a system already running thin. For others, it was environmental: mold in a house they didn't know was sick, heavy metal accumulation, or years of medication that steadily depleted the nutrients their systems depended on.

Sometimes the trigger was sudden. *After that infection, I was never the same. After that pregnancy loss, everything changed. After the mold exposure, I started reacting to everything.* People can often point to a single moment. But the trigger is rarely the whole story. The trigger landed on a system that was already under strain.

Load accumulated. The buffer eroded. And the rules changed.

Why Doing More Makes It Worse

Once the buffer or resilience is gone, the strategy most people reach for, the one that has always worked in every other domain of their life, can often make things worse.

They add more inputs. More supplements. More elimination. More detox protocols. More restriction. More biohacking. The logic feels sound: if something is not working, increase the effort. Refine the approach. Try harder.

But here is what that logic misses: every input requires processing capacity. Supplements must be absorbed through a gut lining, converted by enzymes, detoxified by the liver, and regulated by feedback systems. If the systems responsible for that processing are already strained, if the gut barrier is compromised, detox pathways are overloaded, mitochondria are underperforming, and the nervous system is stuck in a threat state, then adding more inputs does not create more progress. It creates more noise.

This is an argument for targeted supplements rather than untargeted ones. The right supplement, directed at the right system, at the right time, based on what testing has revealed, can be transformative. The problem is not the tool. It is using the tool before you know where to aim it.

I see this regularly in practice. Someone adds methylfolate because they have read about supporting methylation. Within days, they feel worse — more anxious, more wired, sleep deteriorates. The supplement is not wrong. The system receiving it isn't stable enough to process it yet. The input landed on a body that couldn't use it. And instead of building resilience and creating repair, it added demand to a system already operating past its limit.

This is what happens when the body can't process what it is being given. The inputs exceed what the system can handle. Until that processing capacity is restored, stacking untargeted interventions, no matter how well-researched, how well-intentioned, can amplify instability rather than resolve it. The right supplements, aimed at the right system based on what testing reveals, is a different conversation entirely.

Effort without sequence is wasted effort. And this is precisely why intelligent, disciplined people feel worse despite doing everything right. They are applying optimisation strategies to a body that first needs stabilisation. It is like tuning an engine that has no fuel in the tank.

Different Diagnosis. Same Pattern.

This pattern does not belong to one condition.

You see it in autoimmune disease, where the immune system becomes hypervigilant because a compromised gut barrier has blurred the line between threat and normal input. You see it in burnout, where mitochondria can no longer generate consistent energy because the raw materials are depleted and the demand has not stopped. You see it in thyroid dysfunction, where the gland is responding to signals from an unstable system rather than failing on its own. You see it in fertility struggles, where the body has deprioritised reproduction because it doesn't have the resources to sustain it. You see it in chronic gut disorders, in anxiety and mood instability, in mold illness, in accelerated ageing.

Different diagnoses. Same underlying pattern.

In each case, the same pattern played out. The immune system became reactive. The mitochondria became inefficient. Detox pathways slowed. Hormone signaling destabilised. neurotransmitter synthesis downregulated. When the body's capacity to absorb demand runs out, symptoms emerge. Not because the body is broken. Because it is overloaded.

The Question That Changes Everything

When you treat only the symptom, you are treating the signal. Not the source. And suppressing a signal without understanding what generated it is not a solution. It is a delay.

If fatigue persists, the question is not *how do we stimulate more energy?* It is *why is energy production impaired?* If inflammation persists, the question is not *how do we suppress it?* It is *why is the immune system perceiving threat?* If hormones are chaotic, the question is not *how do we override them?* It is *why have these systems lost coordination?*

This is upstream thinking. It is the only way to restore predictability. Because predictability, not perfection, is what real recovery feels like. When your body's responsiveness returns, sleep restores, food tolerance expands, and energy stabilises. Hormones settle. Inflammation quiets. The body responds to what you give it. Effort produces results again.

That is the goal. Not symptom reduction. Getting your body responding again.

But understanding why the body stopped responding is only half the answer. The other half, the half that determines whether understanding translates into recovery, is sequence. Because even knowing what has changed, the order in which you address it matters more than most people realise.

Healing has an order. And that order is not what most people expect.

If this chapter resonated, the Stability Score self-assessment in your workbook will help you identify whether your system currently needs stabilisation, clearing, or optimisation.

The number you land on is your starting point. Everything that follows is designed to move it. *TheHealingHierarchy.com/workbook*

Chapter Three

The Healing Hierarchy: Why Order Creates Outcomes

James had done everything his doctor suggested and most of what his naturopath recommended on top of it.

He was forty-two. He ran a construction business that demanded sixty-hour weeks and a level of mental sharpness he no longer felt he possessed. He had twin toddlers at home. He had not slept a full night in close to three years. He trained when he could, ate well by most standards, and took a handful of supplements that a mate in the wellness space had recommended. He was the kind of man who solved problems by working harder at them, and for most of his life, that approach had delivered results.

But something had changed. The fatigue was no longer the normal tiredness of a busy life. It was a heaviness that didn't lift with rest. Brain fog settled over him mid-morning and stayed. His recovery from training, which used to take a day, now took most of the week. His motivation, something he had never questioned, was draining away. He described it as feeling like he was operating at sixty per cent, all the time, no matter what he did.

His GP ran bloods and found low testosterone. The solution seemed straightforward: testosterone support. He tried it. For a few weeks, something shifted. Energy nudged upward. Then it stalled. The fog returned. The fatigue deepened. He added adaptogens for stress. A

B-vitamin complex. A practitioner-grade magnesium. He reduced his training load. He tried sleeping more, though with twins that was largely theoretical.

Nothing held.

By the time he sat in my clinic, he had a familiar look. Not defeated — frustrated. The look of a man who builds things for a living being told the only explanation was that he was burnt out. He didn't believe it. And he was right not to.

The Right Things in the Wrong Order

James was not doing the wrong things. He was doing them in the wrong order.

His testosterone was genuinely low. But testosterone was not the origin of his problem — it was the consequence. Upstream, his gut was harbouring a Clostridia overgrowth that was producing neurotoxins and draining the very resources his body needed to generate energy and clear waste. His glutathione, the molecule responsible for detoxification at a cellular level, was depleted. His methylation pathways, which govern everything from neurotransmitter production to DNA repair, were impaired. His homocysteine was elevated, a marker that signals the body's processing systems are backed up.

He had been treating the most visible output, the hormone number on the blood test, while the upstream blocks that caused it had never been identified, let alone addressed. It was like repainting the walls of a house while the foundation was cracking. The paint looked fine for a while. Then the cracks came through again.

When we addressed his case in sequence — clearing the gut infection first, restoring detox and methylation capacity second, and only then supporting hormonal signalling — the shift was substantial. Over eight months, his energy returned, the brain fog lifted, and his reliance on caffeine dropped. His testosterone, the number everyone had been chasing from the start, rose significantly, without aggressive hormonal intervention. We had not ignored it. We had addressed what was suppressing it.

His body hadn't been broken — it had been blocked, and the blocks had a sequence.

Healing Has an Order

James's case is one of the most common patterns I see in practice.

The body isn't a flat surface where every intervention carries equal weight. It is a hierarchy. Some systems must stabilise before others can function. Some problems must be cleared before others will respond to treatment. Some interventions, even good ones, even the right ones, will fail or backfire if they are attempted in the wrong order.

I have worked with patients who spent years targeting hormones while their gut was still inflamed. Years supporting adrenal function while foundational nutrient deficiencies went uncorrected. Years optimising supplements while toxins were preventing proper utilisation. They were doing real things. In the wrong order. And the wrong order is why nothing held.

The Healing Hierarchy is a framework for sequencing recovery correctly. It isn't about doing everything at once. It's about knowing what to address first, so that what you do next works. It moves through four levels, and each one creates the conditions for the next.

The Four Levels

The first level is crisis stabilisation, and it is the one most frequently skipped. Before the body can heal, it must be stable enough to begin. If blood sugar is swinging wildly, downstream systems will not settle. If critical nutrient deficiencies are present, for example iron, B12, vitamin D, magnesium, energy production cannot stabilise. If inflammation is acute and active, the body remains locked in survival mode, and survival mode is fundamentally incompatible with repair.

In practice, this is the person whose energy crashes every afternoon, whose sleep fractures at the same hour every night, whose body can't hold a stable baseline long enough for any intervention to take root. Until this layer is addressed, the body is treading water.

The second level is the gut. This surprises many people, particularly those whose primary complaint is fatigue, hormones, or mood. But the gut isn't simply a collection of digestive organs. It governs nutrient absorption, houses the majority of immune activity, influences neurotransmitter production, and communicates directly with the brain through the vagus nerve. If the gut lining is compromised, and in a sensitised system, it very often is, absorption breaks down and chronic immune activation follows. Particles cross the damaged barrier, the immune system responds, and that response drives systemic inflammation affecting mood, thyroid, metabolism, and hormones at once. This is the person taking a full supplement protocol and feeling no different. Not because the supplements are wrong, but because a damaged gut isn't absorbing them. The gut comes second not because symptoms are always digestive, but because gut dysfunction silently undermines every layer above it.

The third level is biochemistry and detox — the body's internal processing capacity. This includes detoxification pathways, methylation, neurotransmitter balance, and cellular energy production. These are the systems responsible for clearing what the body is exposed to, converting nutrients into usable forms, and generating the energy every other function depends on. When these pathways are impaired, the body can't efficiently neutralise toxins, regulate inflammation, or produce stable energy, no matter how clean the diet is or how disciplined the routine.

This is the layer James's case hinged on: his glutathione was depleted, his methylation was impaired, and his detox pathways were backed up. No amount of hormonal support could compensate for a system that had lost its ability to process. This is also why aggressive detox protocols attempted too early often backfire — pushing more material through a blocked system increases symptoms rather than resolving them. When this layer is addressed properly, in sequence, cognitive clarity improves, energy stabilises, and hormonal signalling becomes predictable. The system can process again.

The fourth level is hormones and optimisation. Hormones are often the most visible problem and the place where people most often want to start. But they are rarely the right place to begin. Hormonal signalling depends on stable blood sugar, functional gut absorption, intact detox pathways, and sufficient cellular energy. When those foundations are compromised, hormonal interventions produce inconsistent or short-lived results. This is the woman whose thyroid medication keeps needing adjustment, or the man whose testosterone therapy worked for six weeks and then stopped, because the systems those hormones depend on were never stabilised. When the foundations are restored first, hormonal function often improves significantly without aggressive intervention. Optimisation is the final layer. Not the first.

The sequence is not intuitive. The body's loudest complaint is rarely its deepest problem. And the intervention that feels most urgent is almost never the right place to start.

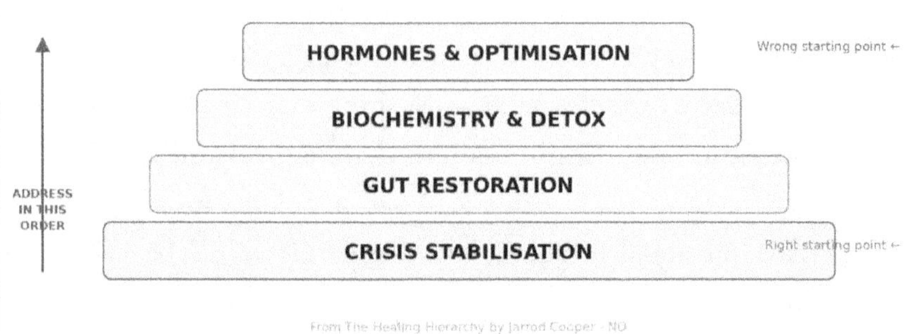

What Gets in the Way

Even when the hierarchy is understood, progress can stall. The sequence may be correct, but something upstream is preventing the body from responding to interventions. I call these Health Blocks.

Health Blocks are upstream burdens that sit beneath the surface, often invisible on basic testing and frequently overlooked:

Gut infections and dysbiosis, bacterial overgrowth, Candida, parasites, and barrier damage generate toxins and immune activation that disrupt every downstream system.

Viral reactivation — Epstein-Barr, CMV, or post-viral syndromes that drain immune and metabolic resources without producing obvious symptoms.

Environmental toxins, mold exposure, heavy metals, and chemical burden increase detox demand beyond what a compromised body can process.

Hidden infections, a lingering dental abscess, and chronic sinus infection can act as a constant low-grade immune trigger that never resolves because nobody thinks to look for it.

Detox and methylation bottlenecks leave the system unable to clear what it is exposed to, no matter how clean the inputs are.

And chronic immune dysregulation, including autoimmune activity, elevated inflammatory markers, and mast cell activation often reflects an unresolved upstream trigger the body has been unable to address on its own.

Health Blocks are not rare edge cases. In a sensitised system, they are common. And they won't resolve on their own. They must be identified and cleared, in the right order, for the hierarchy to deliver results.

Why Protocol Hopping Fails

Most people reading this will recognise the cycle. A new protocol shows promise. There is some improvement — energy lifts, digestion settles, something shifts. Then it plateaus, or new symptoms appear, so they move to the next thing. A different practitioner, a different supplement stack, a different approach. Each one individually reasonable. Each one producing partial or temporary results.

This is not a lack of discipline. It is a predictable outcome of treating downstream symptoms without clearing upstream blocks. If Health Blocks remain active and the hierarchy is ignored, the body can't consolidate gains. Each protocol addresses a piece, but no protocol addresses the sequence. So the pattern repeats. The intervention changes. The outcome does not.

When people say nothing works, what they often mean is this: no one showed them the order in which things *would* work.

Sequence Is the Strategy

James did not need another supplement. He didn't need a new practitioner or a more aggressive hormone protocol. He needed someone to look at his case as a connected system and address it in the right order to stabilise the crisis his body was in. Gut first. Processing capacity second. Hormones last. When that sequence was followed, interventions that had failed before began to hold. His body wasn't resistant to treatment. It had been waiting for the right sequence.

The Healing Hierarchy is not a rigid protocol. It is a decision-making framework. It tells you what to stabilise first, what to repair next, and why the thing you most want to fix may not be the right place to start. It explains why someone can take the right supplement and feel worse, why a hormone intervention can work for six weeks and then fail, and why the person who has tried everything has often tried the right things in the wrong order.

Stability must precede optimisation. Health Blocks must be identified before protocols are layered on top of them. Sequence is the strategy, not a detail of it.

In the chapters ahead, we build the foundation that makes this sequence possible. Because before data can guide decisions, and before interventions can be sequenced, the basics must be in place. Most people overestimate how solid their basics really are.

The hierarchy does not change. Where you enter it does.

In Chapter 17, you will meet Rachel. A woman whose recovery defied this hierarchy because the enemy was not inside her body. It was in her house.

PART II

FOUNDATIONS

Chapter Four

Food as Information

In Chapter 16, you will meet Marcus. Forty-four, lean, disciplined. His diet was textbook — organic, whole food, anti-inflammatory. And it was making him worse. The food was not the issue. His body had lost the ability to process sulfur, histamine, and certain plant compounds that would be harmless in a regulated system. Every 'clean' meal was generating an immune response he could not see and could not override with willpower.

Marcus's story is the advanced version of what this chapter establishes: food is not just nutrition. It is a signal. And when the system receiving that signal is compromised, the quality of the food is not the variable that matters most.

Before we get to Marcus, we need to understand why every meal is a signal.

The meal was simple. Grilled wild caught salmon, steamed broccoli, half a sweet potato, olive oil. By any nutritional standard, it was close to perfect. Nutrient-dense, anti-inflammatory, well-balanced. The kind of meal that appears in every functional medicine textbook as an example of what to eat.

Within ninety minutes, his stomach had bloated to the point of visible distension. Within two hours, the brain fog had settled. By evening, the fatigue had returned in the pattern he had come to dread.

He had not eaten anything wrong. He had eaten something his body could no longer process.

This is where most conversations about diet go wrong: confusing the quality of the food with the capacity of the system receiving it. That is where this chapter begins.

Every Meal Is a Signal

Most conversations about food focus on what it contains: macronutrients, calories, vitamins, fibre. That information matters. But it is only half the picture.

Food is a signal, not just a delivery vehicle for nutrients. Every meal sends instructions to your immune system, your gut bacteria, your hormones, and your blood sugar regulation. A meal high in refined carbohydrates does not just provide glucose. It triggers an insulin response, shifts your microbial environment, and may activate an inflammatory cascade that lasts for hours. A meal built around whole, unprocessed food does the opposite: it stabilises, it nourishes, and it stays quiet.

This is a functional distinction, not a moral one. The same meal that stabilises one person can inflame another. Not because the food is different, but because the body receiving it is. The question is never just *what are you eating?* It is *what is your body doing with what you are eating?* And the answer to that question depends entirely on the state of the system receiving it.

Why Eating Clean Is Not Always Enough

This is where many intelligent, health-conscious people get stuck. They have already removed the obvious offenders. They aren't eating processed food. Yet symptoms persist.

The reason is that food quality and food tolerance are not the same thing. A food can be objectively high quality, nutrient-dense, organic, whole, and still provoke a reaction in a system that has lost its ability to discriminate. When the gut lining is compromised, proteins that should be contained within the digestive tract cross into the bloodstream. The immune system encounters them, registers them as foreign, and mounts a response. That response is inflammation. It can be triggered by foods that are, by any standard, healthy.

This is why someone can react to eggs, almonds, spinach, or bone broth. The food is not the problem. The state of the system receiving it is.

Understanding this distinction changes everything. It means that endlessly restricting your diet without addressing the underlying state of the system becomes a narrowing trap, not a long-term solution. And the path forward is not a smaller food list. It is a more capable body.

Blood Sugar: The Foundation Beneath the Foundation

You know this feeling even if you have never named it. The mid-afternoon crash that arrives no matter what you ate for lunch. The anxiety that appears an hour after a meal and has no obvious cause. The 2 a.m. waking, sudden, wired, inexplicable, that isn't insomnia but a cortisol spike triggered by a blood sugar drop your conscious mind never registered. The irritability. The brain fog that lifts after eating and returns an hour later. These are the sound of unstable blood sugar rippling through every system it touches.

Before addressing food sensitivities, before considering elimination protocols, before anything else — blood sugar must be stable. This is the most underappreciated factor in chronic health conditions, and it is the first thing I address in every case. When blood sugar is volatile, cortisol rises to compensate, the nervous system shifts into a stress response, inflammation increases, and the body's ability to heal is compromised. The fix is structural, not exotic: adequate protein at every meal, sufficient healthy fats, and consistent meal timing.

Stabilising blood sugar is not glamorous. But it is the single most impactful dietary change most people can make, because it reduces the total stress load on the body and creates the conditions for everything else to settle. In the language of the Healing Hierarchy, this is Level 1. For many people, it starts at the table.

The Reset

Once blood sugar is stable, the next step is reducing inflammatory load. Not permanently. Strategically.

A whole food reset strips back to fundamentals: whole, unprocessed foods, quality protein, Healthy fats. Vegetables in abundance. For thirty days, the body gets a break from the inputs most commonly associated with immune activation and inflammatory signalling. The principle is simple: remove the noise and see what settles.

The purpose is not punishment. It is information. When you remove the most common triggers and the bloating eases, the skin clears, the energy stabilises, the brain fog lifts — you have just learned something important. That information is worth more than any food sensitivity test on the market, because it is specific to you, observed in real time, in your body.

I have seen patients whose chronic symptoms resolved within two weeks of a reset. Not because the protocol was magic, but because the inflammatory load was finally low enough for repair to begin. The gut lining started to heal. Immune activation settled. And systems that had been stuck in a reactive state finally had the space to recalibrate.

The reset is the baseline. It is what allows the body to start responding again.

Reintroduction Is the Goal

This is the most important principle in this chapter: elimination is a tool. It isn't an identity.

The purpose of removing foods is not to stay on a restricted diet forever. It is to create a clean baseline from which you can systematically reintroduce foods and observe what your body does with them. One food at a time. Three to four days between introductions. Careful attention to how you feel — energy, digestion, skin, mood, sleep.

Some foods will come back without issue. Others will produce a clear signal: bloating within hours, a skin flare the next morning, fragmented sleep. That food is a food your body can't process right now, in its current state. Once gut integrity improves, once immune activation settles, once the system has more capacity, many of those reactive foods become tolerable again.

The goal is not a smaller and smaller food list. The goal is a body with enough capacity to tolerate a wide variety of real food. My partner Gemma and I have raised six children on this approach. The strict reset for thirty days, followed by an expanded version built for a household of eight that includes real compromises and real meals. It isn't theoretical. And it isn't permanent restriction. Restriction is a temporary strategy. Tolerance is the long-term goal.

The measure of progress is not how disciplined your diet is. It is how much flexibility your body can handle.

When Restriction Becomes the Problem

I see this regularly in practice, and it concerns me more than most things I encounter. People who have been on severely restricted diets for years. Their food list has narrowed to fifteen or twenty items. They are terrified of eating anything outside that list because every reintroduction attempt has produced a reaction. And so they stay. Locked into a pattern that feels safe but is steadily depleting them.

Long-term restriction carries real costs. Nutrient deficiencies accumulate. The gut microbiome loses diversity as the bacteria that thrive on different fibre sources starve. The psychological burden of food fear. The inability to eat at a restaurant, the anxiety about travelling, the social isolation of being unable to share a meal — becomes its own form of stress load.

If your food list keeps shrinking, your system isn't healing.

That is a signal that something upstream needs attention, not a reason to restrict further. The gut lining may still be compromised, an infection may be driving ongoing immune activation, or detox pathways may be overloaded. The diet is managing symptoms, but the underlying state has not changed.

You don't fix food intolerance by removing more food. You fix it by repairing the system that processes food. Gut first. Then the food list takes care of itself.

What Most People Get Wrong

Three mistakes come up again and again.

The first is blaming food when the gut is the real problem. Someone reacts to a food and concludes they are intolerant to it. They may be right, but the intolerance is often a consequence of barrier dysfunction, not a permanent feature of their biology. Removing the food manages the symptom. Repairing the gut resolves the cause.

The second is never reintroducing systematically. People remove foods and never bring them back, or they reintroduce several at once and learn nothing. The reintroduction phase is where the real data lives. Without it, elimination is just restriction with no endpoint.

The third is pursuing dietary perfection at the expense of everything else. I have worked with patients whose diet was immaculate but who were sleeping five hours a night, under enormous stress, and had never addressed a gut infection driving the entire problem. The diet was a ten out of ten. Everything else was a three. And the three was winning.

The goal is not dietary purity. It is physiological resilience. Diet is one foundation among several. And in a sensitised system, the other foundations: sleep, stress, movement, nervous system regulation, often determine whether dietary changes hold.

Food is information. Every meal either supports your body's recovery or adds to its burden. Stabilise blood sugar first, reduce inflammatory load with a reset, and reintroduce systematically. Remember that the goal is a body that can tolerate a wide variety of real food without reacting.

That tolerance is built by restoring the systems that process food, not by restriction alone. And that takes more than what is on your plate.

It also takes sleep.

Chapter Five

Sleep Is Not a Lifestyle Problem

James, the construction company owner you met in Chapter 3, had been waking at 2 a.m. for two years before anyone thought to ask about his sleep. By the time his testosterone crashed and his GP suggested hormone replacement, the damage was already done. Two years of fragmented nights had dismantled his hormonal regulation, his methylation capacity, and his ability to recover from anything.

By the time we restored his sleep architecture, using the principles in this chapter, his testosterone had already begun to climb, before we touched a single hormone. Sleep was not a side issue. It was the upstream driver of everything that followed.

It is 2:17 a.m. and you are awake.

Not the slow, drowsy surfacing of a light sleeper. This is sudden. Sharp. One moment you were asleep. The next you are staring at the ceiling with a heart rate that feels ten beats too fast and a mind already running through tomorrow's obligations. You are tired. You know you need sleep. And you can feel, with the particular frustration of someone who has been through this hundreds of times, that sleep is not coming back.

You have tried everything the articles suggest. The room is dark. The temperature is right. You stopped caffeine after midday. You put the phone down an hour before bed. You took the magnesium. You did the breathing exercise. And here you are, wide awake, wondering what you are doing wrong.

You aren't doing anything wrong. That 2 a.m. waking is not a sleep hygiene failure. It is a cortisol spike — triggered by a blood sugar drop that happened while you were unconscious. Your body registered a crisis, released stress hormones to mobilise glucose, and woke you up as a side effect. The problem is not your bedroom. It is your biochemistry. And until the upstream driver is addressed, no amount of sleep hygiene will fix what is broken.

Sleep Is Not Rest

The word *rest* is misleading. It implies the body is doing nothing, just pausing between productive hours, waiting for morning. The opposite is true. Sleep is the most metabolically active repair state your body enters.

In the first half of the night, deep sleep dominates. This is when the body does its physical repair: growth hormone surges, tissue rebuilds, immune cells are produced, the gut lining restores, and the glymphatic system, designed to wash away metabolic waste, clears inflammatory byproducts that accumulated during waking hours.

In the second half, REM sleep takes over — memory consolidation, emotional processing, hormonal recalibration. If you aren't getting enough of both phases, it's not just fatigue you experience the next day, you are missing the repair cycles that every system in this book depends on.

No supplement compensates for six hours of fragmented sleep. Nothing does.

Gut repair can't happen without adequate sleep, detoxification pathways cannot clear their backlog, and hormone synthesis stalls. Immune regulation loses precision. Every intervention discussed in the chapters ahead: gut protocols, methylation support, hormonal rebalancing, is built on the assumption that the body has a functioning repair window. Sleep is that window. It isn't optional and it isn't replaceable.

Why Sleep Broke

This is the question that matters. The useful question is why the body lost its ability to regulate sleep in the first place.

In a healthy system, sleep regulation is automatic. Cortisol rises in the morning, peaks early, and tapers through the day. By evening, it reaches its lowest point. Melatonin rises in response to dimming light, the nervous system shifts out of its active state, and sleep arrives without effort. You don't have to *try* to sleep. The system handles it.

In a sensitised system, this regulation breaks. And it breaks in predictable ways. When the body has crossed the Sensitization Threshold, sleep is often the first regulatory function to destabilise, and one of the last to fully restore. It is both an early warning that the system is under strain and a bottleneck that prevents recovery until it is addressed.

The most common pattern I see in practice is a cortisol curve that has lost its shape. Instead of peaking in the morning and tapering cleanly, cortisol stays elevated into the evening, or worse, dips during the day when it should be sustaining you and spikes at night when it should be quiet. The result: wired at 11 p.m., exhausted at 7 a.m. Unable to fall asleep despite being tired all day. Or falling asleep without difficulty but waking at 2 or 3 a.m. with no ability to fall back asleep.

This is not insomnia in the classical sense. This is a cortisol regulation problem.

And it is driven by the same upstream factors that drive everything else in this book: blood sugar instability, gut inflammation, chronic immune activation, nervous system dysregulation. The body is stuck in a state of threat, and a body on alert doesn't repair.

The Blood Sugar Connection

Chapter 4 established blood sugar as the foundation beneath the foundation. Nowhere is that more visible than in sleep.

When blood sugar drops during the night, which happens more easily if the evening meal lacked sufficient protein or healthy fats, or if blood sugar regulation is already impaired, the body treats it as a crisis: cortisol is released to mobilise stored glucose, and adrenaline follows. And you wake up: suddenly alert, heart rate elevated, mind racing. It feels like anxiety. It isn't. It is a metabolic rescue response that happens to be incompatible with sleep.

A patient I worked with, a forty-six-year-old project manager, fit, disciplined, eating well by any standard, had been waking between 2 and 3 a.m. almost every night for over two years. She had tried melatonin, magnesium, valerian, a weighted blanket, a sleep restriction protocol, and two different sleep apps. Nothing held for more than a few days. When we reviewed her case, the pattern was clear: her evening meals were low in protein and she was eating dinner at 6 p.m. with nothing after. By 2 a.m., her blood sugar was dropping and her cortisol was spiking to compensate. We added adequate protein to dinner and a small amount of healthy fat before bed. Within three weeks, the 2 a.m. wakings had stopped. Not reduced. Stopped. The problem had never been sleep. It had been fuel.

If you are waking between 2 and 4 a.m. and cannot return to sleep, blood sugar is the first place to look. Before melatonin. Before sleep restriction protocols. Before anything else.

The Clock Beneath the Clock

Your body runs on a circadian rhythm. A roughly twenty-four-hour cycle that governs when cortisol rises, when melatonin is produced, when body temperature drops, when immune activity peaks, and when repair processes activate. This rhythm is calibrated by light. Morning sunlight tells the system it is time to be alert. Dimming light in the evening tells it to prepare for sleep. The cycle repeats, day after day, synchronised with the rotation of the earth.

When this rhythm is intact, sleep is effortless. When it is disrupted, sleep becomes a negotiation.

The most powerful reset I use in practice is the simplest. Ten to fifteen minutes of morning sunlight, as early as possible after waking. Direct light on the face and eyes, not through a window, not through sunglasses. Outside, even in your dressing gown with a cup of tea if that is what it takes. This single habit does more to recalibrate cortisol timing than most supplements, because it is speaking directly to the mechanism that governs the rhythm. It tells the body: *this is morning. Start the clock here.*

At the other end of the day, the signal needs to be equally clear. Blue light from screens, phones, tablets, televisions, laptops, is perceived by the body as daylight. Sitting on your phone at ten o'clock at night is, from your body's perspective, is the same as sitting in the sun. Cortisol responds accordingly. Melatonin production is suppressed. The wind-down that should be happening in the two hours before sleep is replaced by a system that has just been told it is midday.

This isn't a minor lifestyle inconvenience. For someone whose cortisol regulation is already compromised, it is the difference between a system that can find its way back to rhythm and one that can't.

What Sleep Hygiene Can and Cannot Do

Everything you have read about sleep hygiene is probably correct. Cool, dark room, consistent schedule. No caffeine after midday, and if you have anxiety or any sleep difficulty at all, consider removing it entirely. Coffee has a half-life of six hours; half of what you drank at two in the afternoon is still circulating at eight in the evening. Wind down before bed. Reduce screen exposure. These are not myths. They work.

But they work by optimising the environment. They don't fix a system that has lost the ability to function within that environment.

This is the distinction most sleep advice fails to make. If your circadian rhythm is intact, your cortisol curve is healthy, your blood sugar is stable, and your nervous system can shift out of its daytime state, then sleep hygiene is all you need. The environment supports a functioning system.

If any of those upstream regulators are compromised, and in a sensitised body, several usually are, then sleep hygiene becomes necessary but is not enough. You can have the perfect bedroom and still lie awake, because the system that converts environmental cues into sleep is not functioning. The cues are present. The translator is broken.

This is why I address sleep on two levels. The hygiene layer: environment, light, temperature, timing, stimulant management. Then the regulatory layer: blood sugar stabilisation, cortisol rhythm restoration, nervous system support, and addressing whatever upstream load is preventing the system from settling. The hygiene creates the conditions. The regulatory work restores the body's ability to use them.

Bridges, Not Replacements

Patients ask me about sleep supplements constantly. Magnesium, melatonin, GABA, 5-HTP, L-theanine, passionflower, valerian. Some of these have genuine utility. Magnesium glycinate before bed supports muscle relaxation and nervous system calming. L-theanine can ease the transition out of an active mind state. Low-dose melatonin can be helpful over shorter periods for circadian rhythm resetting, particularly after travel or shift work.

But these are bridges. They aren't solutions. A bridge gets you across a gap while the road is being rebuilt. It doesn't replace the road. If you are relying on a supplement to sleep and the moment you stop taking it the problem returns, the supplement is managing a symptom. The upstream driver. The cortisol dysregulation, the blood sugar instability, the nervous system stuck in overdrive, has not been addressed.

The goal is a body that can fall asleep and stay asleep without pharmaceutical or nutraceutical assistance. Supplements are not the problem, but needing them to sleep signals that something upstream has not been resolved. The exception is magnesium glycinate. It is a foundational nutrient, not a sleep aid. Most people are deficient. Long-term supplementation is appropriate and benefits far more than just sleep. Use them while you need them. But if you cannot sleep without a supplement, that is not a solution. That is information. Something upstream is still unresolved.

The Non-Negotiable

Eight hours of sleep between 10 p.m. and 6 a.m. is not the same physiological event as eight hours between 2 a.m. and 10 a.m. The body's deepest physical repair - growth hormone release, immune restoration, tissue rebuilding - concentrates in the early sleep cycles, which are richest when you fall asleep earlier in the evening. The later cycles are dominated by REM sleep, where emotional processing, memory consolidation, and hormonal recalibration occur. Go to bed too late and you lose deep sleep. Wake too early and you lose REM. If you are habitually going to bed at midnight or later, you are shortchanging the repair cycles your body depends on. You will feel it in recovery, in inflammation, in the speed at which your body responds to treatment.

I am direct with every patient on this point: if you aren't sleeping seven to eight hours, in a pattern broadly aligned with the earth's light and dark cycle, every other intervention in this book will underperform. Sleep is not one factor among many. It is the repair window that everything else depends on.

If you work shifts, perfect alignment with the light-dark cycle may not be possible, but the principles still apply. Consistent sleep timing, morning light exposure on waking regardless of the hour, and protecting your longest unbroken sleep window become even more critical. Work with what you have, not against it.

I have had patients rework their sleep patterns from 2 a.m. bedtimes back to 10 p.m. within a matter of weeks. It doesn't require medication. It requires resetting the circadian clock: morning sunlight, consistent wake times, evening light reduction, and addressing whatever is preventing the body from winding down. For some, that is blood sugar. For others, it is cortisol. For others, it is a gut infection producing neurotoxins that keep the nervous system activated. The entry point varies. The principle does not.

Food stabilises the system. Sleep repairs it. But there is a third foundation that most people in this state get wrong. Not because they are inactive, but because they are doing the wrong kind of activity at the wrong time. For a body that has crossed the Sensitization Threshold, movement is not what most people think it is.

It is a signal. And the signal matters more than the sweat.

Chapter Six

Movement Without Drain

In Chapter 12, you will meet Emma. Thirty-nine, Hashimoto's thyroiditis, and a history of pushing through. She had always trained hard. It was how she managed stress, maintained her weight, and held onto her identity during years of declining health. When her thyroid antibodies climbed and her energy collapsed, her instinct was to train harder. It made everything worse.

Emma's recovery required a period where rest was the protocol and movement was carefully matched to her system's actual capacity. Not the capacity she remembered. That principle is what this chapter teaches, and it applies whether you are managing an autoimmune condition or simply noticing that your body no longer recovers the way it used to.

She had always been someone who moved. Running in her twenties. CrossFit in her thirties. By forty-one, she had dialled it back to three strength sessions and two HIIT classes a week. A programme that would be considered balanced by any standard. Training was structure, stress relief, identity. It was the thing she could count on when nothing else cooperated.

Then it stopped cooperating too.

Recovery times stretched. A session that used to leave her energised now left her flattened for two days. She pushed through it, because that is what she had always done. The fatigue deepened, her sleep fragmented, and her joints ached in ways they never had. She reduced volume. She reduced intensity. She rested more. And then she noticed something that frightened her: on the days she rested completely, she felt worse. On the days she trained, she crashed the next morning. There was no version of movement that didn't cost her something she could not afford.

By the time she sat in my clinic, she had already drawn her own conclusion: her body could no longer tolerate exercise. She was wrong. Her body couldn't tolerate the signal that exercise was sending.

Movement Is a Signal

Most people think about exercise in terms of output. Calories burned. Distance covered. Weight lifted. Sets completed. By that logic, more is always better — more volume, more intensity, more consistency. In a healthy, regulated body, that logic broadly holds. You train, you stress the system, the system adapts, and you come back stronger. The stress is productive.

But exercise is not just an output. It is an input. Every session sends a signal to your nervous system, your hormones, your immune function, and your metabolic machinery. A moderate walk in the morning tells the nervous system: *you are safe. The environment is stable. Resources can be directed toward repair.* A high-intensity interval session tells it something very different: *this is a threat. Mobilise cortisol, divert resources to survival, and shut down non-essential processes.*

In a resilient body, the threat signal is temporary. You train hard. Cortisol rises, then falls. Recovery begins. The system absorbs the stress and adapts. That is how fitness is built.

In a sensitised body, one that has crossed the Sensitization Threshold, the threat signal does not resolve. Cortisol rises and stays elevated. The nervous system, already stuck in a stress state, receives confirmation that the threat is real. Recovery is delayed or incomplete, inflammation increases, and sleep fragments. The training session that was supposed to build you up has instead drained you. The signal matters more than the sweat.

When Exercise Becomes a Stressor

Exercise is a controlled dose of stress that stimulates adaptation. Too much breaks you down and the body can't recover. Too little, and the body deconditions. The dose is everything. The therapeutic window, the range in which exercise builds capacity without exceeding recovery, depends entirely on the state of the system receiving it.

In a healthy system, that window is wide. You can train hard, recover quickly, and adapt. In a sensitised system, the window narrows dramatically. What used to be a moderate session is now an excessive demand. What used to produce adaptation now produces a crash.

I see this pattern constantly in practice. Someone who used to train five days a week, no issues, is now unable to recover from a forty-minute strength session. They assume they are unfit. They assume they need to push harder. So they do, and the crash that follows is worse than the one before. Every small improvement is followed by a setback. They describe it as two steps forward, three steps back. The instinct to push through, the instinct that has served them in every other area of life, is the very thing making it worse.

Pushing through is not discipline. In a sensitised body, it is a strategy that backfires every time.

High-intensity training in particular can stall healing. It raises cortisol in a system that already can't clear cortisol efficiently. It increases metabolic demand on mitochondria that are already underperforming. It diverts resources away from immune regulation, gut repair, and detoxification. The very processes the body needs to recover. The problem is not the exercise. It is the mismatch between the demand of the session and the capacity of the system absorbing it.

What Actually Builds Resilience

If high-intensity training can drain a sensitised system, what builds it back?

Three things, in order of priority: walking, strength training, and low-intensity aerobic work.

Walking is the most underrated form of movement in health recovery, and it is the one I prescribe most often. It pumps the lymphatic system, the body's waste removal network, which has no pump of its own and relies on movement to circulate. It exposes you to natural light, which supports circadian rhythm and vitamin D production. It activates the parasympathetic nervous system without elevating cortisol. And it does all of this without asking the body for anything it can't afford to give.

Thirty minutes of walking per day, ideally outside, ideally in the morning, is more therapeutically valuable for someone in a sensitised state than any gym session.

Strength training is the second priority, and it matters for reasons that go well beyond aesthetics. Muscle is metabolic currency. It is the primary site where your body disposes of glucose, which means more muscle mass directly improves insulin sensitivity and blood sugar regulation. The very foundation we established in Chapter 4. Muscle mass is also one of the strongest predictors of resilience as you age. It protects bone density. It supports hormonal signalling. It maintains the functional movement patterns: squatting, lunging, hinging, pushing, pulling, rotating, that keep the body capable and injury-resistant through life.

But in a sensitised system, the approach matters as much as the activity. Two to three sessions per week, moderate load, controlled tempo, Adequate rest between sets. The point isn't to destroy the muscle and hope it rebuilds. It's to stimulate adaptation without exceeding recovery capacity. You should leave a strength session feeling like you worked, not like you need to lie down. If you can't recover from a session within twenty-four hours, the intensity or volume is too high for your current state.

The third element is Zone 2 cardio — low-intensity aerobic work at a pace where you can hold a conversation comfortably. It doesn't feel hard. It should not feel hard. That is the point. At this intensity, your body preferentially burns fat for fuel, builds mitochondrial density, and improves the efficiency of cellular energy production. The very machinery that is underperforming in a sensitised system. Zone 2 work builds the engine without overloading it. Walking counts. Cycling at an easy pace counts. Swimming laps without pushing counts. The threshold is simple: if you can't talk in full sentences, you are working too hard for where your body is right now.

Matching Movement to Your State

This is the principle that most exercise advice ignores: the right movement depends on the state of the body performing it. There is no universally correct exercise programme. There is only what your current capacity can absorb and benefit from.

If you are actively healing, your symptoms are present, your recovery is slow, and your energy is unpredictable, prioritise walking and gentle movement daily, with two to three light strength sessions per week. This is matching the dose to the capacity. The body can't build new resilience while it is still trying to stabilise.

If you are stabilising - symptoms are settling, sleep is improving, energy is becoming more consistent - you can begin to add volume. Zone 2 cardio two to three times per week. Progressive overload in strength work, gradually. This is where the body begins to adapt again. But the key word is gradually. The temptation at this stage is to rush back to previous training levels. Do not. The system that crashed once is more vulnerable to crashing again if the ramp-up is too aggressive.

If you are optimising - symptoms are resolved, energy is stable, recovery is functioning normally - the window opens. Higher-intensity work becomes appropriate. Intervals. VO_2 max training (training at 90-100% of your maximum heart rate). Progressive overload with real intent. This is where performance goals become realistic again. But even here, recovery must be monitored. The body that has crossed the Threshold and come back carries a deeper understanding of what happens when demand exceeds capacity. That understanding is an asset, not a limitation.

When Rest Is the Protocol

There is a version of this conversation that is harder than the rest. It is the one I have with patients who are crashing — whose fatigue is so deep that a fifteen-minute walk leaves them spent for the rest of the day. Whose bodies respond to any form of exertion with disproportionate exhaustion that lasts days rather than hours.

For these patients, rest is not laziness. Rest is the intervention.

This is counterintuitive for people who have built their identity on discipline and effort. Being told to rest feels like surrender. But forcing movement on a body that cannot recover from it is not discipline. It is damage. The system needs to rebuild enough baseline stability to tolerate gentle movement before movement can become therapeutic. Pushing through before that baseline exists extends the recovery timeline. Every time.

The goal isn't permanent rest. It's strategic rest — enough to allow the foundations to stabilise, so that when movement is reintroduced, the body can actually use it. Blood sugar must be stable. Sleep must be functional. The nervous system must have enough capacity to shift out of its threat state. Once those conditions are met, walking is reintroduced. Then gentle strength work. Then, gradually, the window opens.

The woman from the beginning of this chapter followed this path. She stopped training entirely for six weeks, walked daily, and stabilised her blood sugar and her sleep. Then reintroduced two light strength sessions per week, with no conditioning work. Within three months, she was training three times a week without crashing, not at her previous intensity, but with genuine enjoyment and without the two-day recovery debt that had made movement feel impossible. The body doesn't forget how to move. It needs the conditions to be able to move again.

The Movement Most People Miss

One thing I emphasise with every patient: movement extends beyond gym work to how you use your body through the day. The functional movement patterns: squatting, lunging, hinging, pushing, pulling, rotating, and walking under load, are the movements your body was designed for. They keep joints mobile, muscles balanced, and the nervous system communicating properly with the musculoskeletal system.

You only have to look at a child to understand this. A two-year-old can sit in a deep squat for twenty minutes, flat-footed, spine neutral, completely at ease. Most adults cannot hold that position for thirty seconds. That is not ageing. That is the accumulation of sitting, poor posture, restricted range, and movement patterns that were never maintained. If you don't use it, you lose it. And when you lose functional movement, the body compensates — loading joints and muscles in ways they weren't designed for, which leads to pain, injury, and further restriction.

The nervous system plays a role here that most people do not appreciate. When there is high inflammation, chronic stress, or neural tension, the body will shut down range of movement to protect itself. Muscles that should fire do not. Compensation patterns develop. You go to do a deadlift and your glutes do not activate, so your lower back takes the load. Injury follows. The solution is not to push harder. It is to reduce the underlying inflammation and stress that is causing the nervous system to restrict movement in the first place, and then retrain the functional patterns.

The right movement at the right time strengthens you. The wrong movement at the wrong time sets you back.

Food stabilises. Sleep repairs. Movement builds. These three foundations form a single integrated base. When all three are aligned with what the body needs, recovery has a platform to build on. When any one of them is mismatched, too much food, not enough sleep, wrong type of movement, the platform is unstable and everything layered on top of it underperforms.

But there is a fourth element that sits beneath all three. It determines how the body processes food, how deeply it sleeps, and whether movement builds or drains. It is not a behaviour. It is the nervous system. And in a sensitised body, it is almost always dysregulated.

The nervous system. And learning to work with it, not override it, is where the shift begins.

A basic functional movement guide covering the key patterns for building strength and resilience without exceeding recovery capacity, is available at TheHealingHierarchy.com

Movement is medicine. But the dose must match the capacity that is available at the time.

Chapter Seven

The Nervous System Is Not a Mindset Problem

In Chapter 13, you will meet Alex. Twenty-one, university student, with crippling anxiety that appeared from nowhere. His GP prescribed an SSRI to assist with his seratonin. It made him emotionally numb. University counselling taught stress management techniques. They helped with the thoughts but not the physical symptoms. The racing heart, the chest tightness, the three-hour wait to fall asleep every night.

Alex's anxiety was not a mind problem. It was a brain problem with a biochemical cause. But the starting point of his recovery was his nervous system. Until his body could shift out of the threat state it had been locked in for eighteen months, no intervention we used would hold. This chapter explains why, and what to do about it.

I can usually tell within the first ten minutes of a consultation whether someone's nervous system is stuck. Not because the signs are dramatic — they rarely are. The person sitting across from me may be composed, articulate, and entirely reasonable. But their body tells a different story. Their shoulders are braced. Their breathing is shallow — short, quick breaths that barely reach the chest, let alone the diaphragm. They speak quickly, as if running out of time even when there is plenty. When I ask about sleep, digestion, or recovery, the pattern is consistent: everything is reactive, nothing is settling, and the harder they try, the worse it gets.

They have often been told to relax. To meditate. To think more positively. To manage their stress. They have tried — genuinely, repeatedly, sometimes for years. The advice has not worked. Not because they are doing it wrong. But because the advice misunderstands the problem.

Stress is a nervous system response, not a mindset failure. You can't think your way out of a body that is stuck on high alert.

Two Modes, One Body

Your autonomic nervous system, the part of your nervous system that operates below conscious control, runs in two primary modes. The sympathetic branch is your threat response: fight, flight, freeze. It elevates cortisol, increases heart rate, diverts blood away from digestion and toward the muscles, sharpens focus, and mobilises energy. It is designed to keep you alive in a crisis. When it activates, every non-essential process is deprioritised: digestion slows, immune regulation is suppressed and tissue repair is deferred. Hormone production shifts to favour survival over reproduction or recovery.

The parasympathetic branch is the opposite state: rest, digest, repair. It lowers cortisol, slows the heart rate, restores blood flow to the digestive organs, activates immune surveillance, and opens the repair window that sleep, food, and movement depend on. This is the state in which the body heals. Not the only state, but the essential one.

In a healthy system, these two branches alternate fluidly. You encounter a stressor, the sympathetic branch activates, the stressor passes, and the parasympathetic branch takes over to restore balance. The transition is automatic. You don't have to do anything to make it happen.

In a sensitised system, the transition stops happening.

In a sensitised system, the sympathetic branch activates in response to a stressor and stays activated. Long after the threat has passed, the body remains in threat mode. Not because the person is anxious or thinking negative thoughts. Because the nervous system has simply lost the ability to shift back. It is stuck. While it is stuck, every other system in the body is operating under threat conditions: reduced digestion, elevated inflammation, suppressed immune function, disrupted hormone signalling, and impaired repair.

This is why someone can do everything right: eat perfectly, sleep eight hours, take every supplement in the protocol, and still not improve. The inputs are correct. But the system receiving them is in the wrong state to use them. You can't digest food efficiently in sympathetic dominance. You can't repair tissue in fight-or-flight. You can't regulate hormones when the body believes it is under attack.

The body must feel safe before it can heal. Safety is not a thought. It is a neurological state.

Why the System Got Stuck

The nervous system doesn't get stuck because of one bad week at work. It gets stuck because of cumulative, unresolved load. The same pattern that drives everything else in this book.

Blood sugar instability is one of the most common and most overlooked drivers. Every time blood sugar crashes, the body releases cortisol to compensate. In someone eating irregularly, skipping meals, or relying on refined carbohydrates, this can happen multiple times per day — each spike reinforcing the threat state. The nervous system doesn't distinguish between a blood sugar crisis and a physical danger. It responds the same way. This is why the dietary foundation in Chapter 4 matters so much: stabilising blood sugar removes one of the most persistent triggers keeping the nervous system locked.

Chronic psychological stress compounds the nervous system dysregulation. But so do sources the person may not recognise as stress at all. Gut infections produce inflammatory signals that activate the sympathetic branch, independently of anything happening in your life. Sleep deprivation impairs the nervous system's ability to reset overnight. Environmental toxins, food sensitivities, and chronic immune activation all maintain the threat state through persistent inflammatory signalling.

Telling someone to 'just relax' isn't just unhelpful. It misunderstands the biology. Relaxation is something the nervous system produces when conditions allow, not something you can impose on it. If the system can't shift because of upstream inflammation, blood sugar crises, gut-derived toxins, or chronic immune activation, then no amount of willpower will produce relaxation. You are asking the body to do something it currently cannot do.

The Fastest Tool You Have

Of all the inputs that can shift nervous system state, breath is the most immediate and the most accessible.

The diaphragm is a muscle, and in most people I see in practice, it is barely used. Shallow, chest-level breathing is a hallmark of chronic sympathetic activation. The body breathes as if it is preparing for threat: short, quick, upper-chest breaths that keep the system primed. Most people do not notice they are doing it. It has become their baseline.

Deliberate, structured breathing overrides this. When you extend the exhale beyond the inhale, you directly stimulate the vagus nerve, the primary communication pathway between the brain and the body's organs. The vagus nerve is the parasympathetic highway. Stimulating it sends a direct signal to the brain: *the threat has passed. Begin recovery. Heart rate drops, cortisol begins to clear, digestion reactivates*. The repair window opens.

This is measurable physiology. A single session of structured breathing can shift heart rate variability, one of the most reliable markers of nervous system state, within minutes. Not hours. Not weeks. Minutes. No supplement acts that fast. No dietary change acts that fast. Breath is the fastest lever you have for changing the state of your nervous system.

I worked with a woman in her late thirties. A teacher, mother of two, presenting with chronic fatigue, irritable bowel symptoms, and anxiety that had appeared seemingly from nowhere. Her bloods were unremarkable, her diet was excellent, and she was sleeping seven hours. Every conventional and functional marker looked reasonable. But her breathing pattern was telling: fourteen to eighteen breaths per minute at rest, all in the upper chest. A healthy resting rate is ten to twelve. Her nervous system had been running in threat mode for so long that she no longer recognised it as abnormal. We started with five minutes of box breathing, four seconds in, four seconds hold, four seconds out, four seconds hold, twice daily. Within three weeks, her IBS symptoms had reduced by half. Not because the breathing fixed her gut. But because the nervous system shift allowed her gut to function again.

Breath as Practice

I recommend breath work to almost every patient. Not as a wellness add-on. As a clinical tool.

The simplest protocol is box breathing: four seconds inhale, four seconds hold, four seconds exhale, four seconds hold. Four rounds. Twice daily — morning and evening. It takes five minutes total. It is structured enough to override habitual shallow breathing and long enough to produce a measurable shift in nervous system tone. For patients with significant anxiety or sleep difficulty, the 4-7-8 pattern is more effective: four seconds inhale, seven seconds hold, eight seconds exhale. The extended exhale drives a stronger parasympathetic response. Fill the diaphragm first then the top lungs. Relax the shoulders. Push out as much air as possible at the end of the exhale.

The Wim Hof method, a series of rapid, deep breaths followed by extended breath holds, works differently. It is more activating, not calming. It trains the body's tolerance to stress by deliberately inducing a controlled stress response and then recovering from it. This builds resilience over time. But it isn't appropriate for everyone, particularly those whose nervous systems are deeply stuck in sympathetic dominance. For those patients, calming protocols come first. Resilience training comes later, once the baseline has shifted.

The pattern from the previous chapters holds: match the tool to the state. If you are stuck in threat mode, the priority is calming the system. If you are stabilising, you can begin to train resilience. The breath work should feel like it is helping, not like it is another demand on a depleted body.

Cold Exposure: The Right Tool at the Right Time

Cold exposure is one of the most powerful tools available for improving resilience, mood, and metabolic function. A single session of cold-water immersion has been shown to increase dopamine by 250 percent and norepinephrine by 530 percent, with effects lasting up to two hours. Those are not small numbers. For context, norepinephrine is the same neurotransmitter targeted by SNRI medications prescribed for depression and anxiety. Cold water can produce a comparable neurochemical shift without a prescription.

But here is where I need to be honest with you, because this is where most health books and most practitioners get it wrong.

Cold exposure is a hormetic stressor. It works by deliberately stressing the body and allowing it to recover stronger. That is the definition of hormesis: a small, controlled dose of stress that triggers an adaptive response. Exercise is hormesis. Fasting is hormesis. And cold exposure is hormesis.

The key word in that definition is *recover*.

Hormesis only works if your body has the capacity to recover from the stress. If it does not, the stress is not hormetic. It is just stress. And stress, applied to a system that is already overwhelmed, does not make you stronger. It makes you worse.

This is the Healing Hierarchy in action.

If you are reading this book, there is a high probability that your HPA axis — your hypothalamic-pituitary-adrenal axis, the system that governs your stress response, is dysregulated. In chronic illness, particularly in chronic fatigue, autoimmune conditions, and long-term inflammatory states, the HPA axis is frequently disrupted. Cortisol rhythms flatten. The normal morning peak disappears. The body loses its ability to mount an appropriate stress response and then return to baseline.

Now picture what happens when you step into an ice bath.

Your sympathetic nervous system activates immediately. Adrenaline surges. Norepinephrine floods your system. Heart rate spikes. Blood pressure rises. Peripheral blood vessels constrict. Your body enters a full fight-or-flight response.

For a healthy person with a well-regulated HPA axis, this is a controlled challenge. The body mounts the stress response, rides the wave, and returns to baseline stronger than before. That is hormesis working as intended.

For someone whose HPA axis is already dysregulated - whose cortisol is already flattened, whose nervous system is already stuck in sympathetic dominance, whose adrenals are already running on empty. This becomes another hit to a system that can't absorb it. You are adding acute stress to a body that hasn't recovered from chronic stress. The stress response fires, but the recovery does not follow. You feel terrible. You crash. Your sleep worsens. Your inflammation increases. And you wonder why something that is supposed to be good for you made you worse.

The answer is not that cold exposure is bad. The answer is that it was the right tool at the wrong time.

This is exactly the pattern I see in clinic, again and again. A patient has been told that ice baths are anti-inflammatory. They are. She has been told they boost the immune system. They do. She has been told they improve mood and energy. They can. But nobody told her that those benefits are only available to a body that has the physiological capacity to mount and recover from the stress response that cold exposure demands. Nobody told her where cold exposure sits in the hierarchy.

Cold exposure belongs in the later stages of recovery. It is a Level 4 intervention. It isn't where you start. If your HPA axis is dysregulated, if your cortisol rhythm is disrupted, if your sleep is broken, if your nervous system is locked in sympathetic overdrive - cold exposure is not your next step. Restoring nervous system regulation is your next step. Rebuilding your circadian rhythm is your next step. Stabilising your HPA axis is your next step. Cold exposure earns its place after that foundation is in place.

Cold Exposure Is Not the Same for Women and Men

There is another problem with the way cold exposure is currently promoted, and it is one that affects the majority of my patients directly.

Almost everything you have heard about ice baths comes from research conducted on men, promoted by men, and optimised for male physiology. The Wim Hof protocols. The Andrew Huberman recommendations. The social media clips of men sitting in tubs of ice at two degrees Celsius and telling you to push through the discomfort. That works for male physiology. It doesn't work the same way for female physiology.

Women respond differently to cold exposure than men. Research from Dr Stacy Sims and Dr Susanna Søeberg has shown that when women are exposed to extreme cold, the same intense stress response that produces beneficial adaptations in men can overshoot in women - elevating cortisol, suppressing thyroid activity, and blunting the hormonal and metabolic benefits the cold exposure was supposed to produce.

Women reach shivering thresholds earlier. Women report cold more intensely at warmer temperatures. Women have higher core body temperatures at baseline, which means the thermal shock of extreme cold is proportionally greater. And women's hormonal cycles add another variable for which male-based protocols simply do not account. During the luteal phase of the menstrual cycle, sensitivity to temperature changes increases, and shorter, warmer exposures are more appropriate.

The emerging consensus from female-specific research is clear: women benefit from cold exposure at warmer temperatures and shorter durations than the protocols popularised on social media. The optimal range for most women is fourteen to fifteen degrees Celsius (fifty-seven to fifty-nine degrees Fahrenheit) for two to five minutes. That is not an ice bath. That is cool water immersion. And the difference matters.

Stanford's Dr Anna Lembke, one of the leading researchers on dopamine and addiction, recommends graded exposure for all patients: start with warmer temperatures and shorter durations, and observe each person's individual response. She has noted that some patients with chronic pain and mental health conditions reacted negatively to cold exposure and were advised to either discontinue or reduce the dose significantly.

I agree with this approach entirely. There is no single temperature or duration that is right for everyone. Your body will tell you. If you feel energised and alert after cold exposure, the dose is right. If you feel wired, anxious, exhausted, or you crash later in the day, the dose is too high or the timing is wrong.

A Practical Framework

Before introducing cold exposure into your recovery, ask yourself these questions:

- Is my sleep consistently restorative? Am I waking rested?

- Is my cortisol rhythm normalising? Am I alert in the morning and tired at night?

- Am I out of sympathetic dominance? Can I rest without feeling wired?

- Is my HPA axis function stabilising based on testing?

- Have I addressed the foundational levels of the Healing Hierarchy first?

If the answer to any of these is no, cold exposure is not your next step. Work on the foundations first. Cold exposure will still be there when you are ready for it. When you are ready, it will work far better because your body will have the capacity to respond to it properly.

When you are ready, use this as a starting framework:

Entry level — eighteen to twenty degrees Celsius. A cool shower at the end of a warm shower, thirty to sixty seconds. Minimal sympathetic stress. Safe starting point for anyone in recovery.

Women, stabilised — fourteen to fifteen degrees Celsius for two to five minutes. This is the range supported by female-specific research. Activates brown fat and cold thermogenesis while maintaining parasympathetic balance. Bias warmer and shorter during the luteal phase. Some women will tolerate colder over time, but progress based on cycle phase and recovery, not comparison to male protocols.

Men, stabilised — ten to fourteen degrees Celsius for two to five minutes. Standard hormetic zone for male physiology. Produces robust metabolic adaptations, brown fat activation, and neurotransmitter release. Once you're stable in this range, you can push colder — but the adaptation should be earned, not forced.

Extreme (social media protocols) — two to four degrees Celsius. Not recommended for chronic illness recovery. Disproportionate stress load. Risk of cold shock, after-drop, and HPA axis disruption. This is performance dosing, not healing.

Start at the entry level. Stay there for at least two weeks. If you feel good, actually good, not just endorphin-high good, move to the next level. If you feel worse at any point, go back a level or stop entirely. There is no failure in deciding that cold exposure is not right for you at this stage of your recovery. There is only the intelligence to recognise that your body is telling you something and the discipline to listen to it.

Cold exposure is a remarkable tool — I use it myself and recommend it to patients regularly. But I recommend it at the right time, at the right dose, and with an understanding that what works for a healthy thirty-year-old man training for performance is not the same as what works for a woman recovering from years of chronic illness. The Healing Hierarchy applies here just as it applies everywhere else in this book. Sequence matters. Foundation first.

Heat Exposure as Nervous System Training

Infrared saunas work the other end of the spectrum. Unlike traditional steam saunas, infrared heat penetrates tissue directly, promoting circulation, supporting detoxification, and producing a deep parasympathetic relaxation response. Twenty to forty-five minutes, two to four times per week, is a protocol I recommend for patients who tolerate it well. Heat exposure is generally better tolerated than cold exposure for patients in the earlier stages of recovery because it supports parasympathetic activation rather than demanding a sympathetic stress response.

The Nerve That Connects Everything

The vagus nerve deserves its own attention, because it is the physical infrastructure that connects the nervous system to everything else in this book.

It runs from the brainstem through the neck and into the chest and abdomen, branching into the heart, lungs, liver, stomach, and intestines. It carries signals in both directions: from the brain to the organs, and from the organs back to the brain. Approximately ninety-five percent of serotonin, the neurotransmitter most associated with mood regulation, is produced in the gastrointestinal tract. The vagus nerve is the pathway through which that gut-produced serotonin communicates with the brain.

This is the biological mechanism behind the gut-brain connection. When the gut is inflamed, the vagus nerve carries that inflammatory signal to the brain, which interprets it as threat. When the brain perceives threat, it sends sympathetic signals back through the vagus nerve, further suppressing digestion. The loop reinforces itself: gut dysfunction drives nervous system activation, which drives further gut dysfunction. Breaking the loop requires working on both ends at once — clearing the gut, and calming the nervous system.

Vagal tone, the strength of the vagus nerve's parasympathetic signalling, can be improved. Breath work is the most direct method. But singing, humming, and gargling also stimulate the vagus nerve through the muscles of the throat. Cold exposure activates it powerfully. These are direct physiological interventions that strengthen the parasympathetic pathway.

The nervous system doesn't care what you know. It responds to what it feels.

When the Nervous System Becomes the Problem

Everything in this chapter so far has addressed the nervous system as a consequence, something that gets stuck because upstream drivers are keeping it locked. Blood sugar instability, gut inflammation, chronic immune activation, environmental toxins. Remove those drivers, and the nervous system settles. For most patients, that is exactly what happens. The threat signal fades as the upstream load reduces. The body shifts back into repair mode. Recovery accelerates.

But not always.

There is a subset of patients I see where the upstream work has been done. The gut is repaired. The infections are cleared. The biochemistry is improving. The labs are heading in the right direction. And yet the nervous system remains locked. They still react to foods that should no longer be a problem. They still cannot tolerate supplements they should be able to handle. Sleep is still fragile. The body still behaves as though it is under threat, even when the data says the threat has been addressed.

This is not a failure of the protocol. It is a different problem. The nervous system has learned to be in threat mode. And the learning has become self-sustaining.

The brain is not a fixed structure. It is plastic, constantly rewiring itself based on repeated input, a property called neuroplasticity. When a nervous system has been locked in a threat response for months or years, those neural pathways become deeply reinforced. The brain gets faster and more efficient at producing the threat response, because that is the pattern it has been practising. At some point, the original trigger becomes irrelevant. The pattern itself becomes the trigger. A symptom appears, the brain interprets it as confirmation of ongoing danger, the nervous system activates, more symptoms follow, and the cycle reinforces itself. The loop runs on its own.

I have seen this in patients whose recovery stalls at seventy or eighty per cent. Their test results have improved. Their protocols are sound. They are doing the work. But their bodies remain hypervigilant, reacting to supplements that should help, flaring from foods they have successfully reintroduced before, unable to expand their tolerance despite the underlying systems improving. When I see this pattern, objective improvement on paper but subjective stagnation in the body, the nervous system is almost always the remaining piece.

Recognising this matters, because the treatment approach is different. You do not fix a conditioned nervous system by running more tests or adding more supplements. You fix it by retraining the brain.

Neuroplasticity works in both directions. The same mechanism that allowed the threat response to become entrenched can be used to dismantle it. The brain can learn a new pattern, one where safety replaces threat as the default. This is not positive thinking. It is not pushing through symptoms. It is structured, repeated practice that teaches the nervous system a different response to the signals it is receiving.

In practice, this looks like deliberate interruption of the threat loop. When a symptom appears and the familiar cascade of fear, monitoring, and bracing begins, the patient learns to consciously redirect the response. Not by ignoring the symptom, but by changing what the brain does with it. Over time, with consistent practice, the brain builds a new pathway. Symptom appears. Recognition without alarm. The nervous system stays calm. The symptom resolves faster because the body is not amplifying it with a stress response. The old pathway does not disappear overnight. But it weakens as the new one strengthens. That is neuroplasticity.

There are structured programs designed specifically for this work, and some of my patients have found them transformative, particularly those with multiple chemical sensitivities, chronic fatigue that persists after treatment, or food reactivity that does not match their test results. I do not prescribe a specific program, because the right approach depends on the individual. But the principle is consistent: the nervous system must be retrained, not just calmed.

The tools earlier in this chapter, breathwork, cold exposure, vagal stimulation, remain essential. They create the conditions for retraining by giving the nervous system repeated experiences of shifting out of threat mode. But for patients whose pattern has become deeply conditioned, those tools are the foundation, not the finish line. The finish line is a brain that no longer defaults to threat in the absence of an actual threat.

Here is how I think about it clinically. If a patient is improving on paper but not in their body, I ask three questions.

First: are there upstream drivers we have missed? A hidden infection, an undiagnosed mold exposure, a dental issue, something still generating a legitimate threat signal.

Second: is the protocol correct but the timing wrong? Some interventions need more time to produce a felt result than the data suggests.

And third: has the nervous system become self-sustaining? Has the pattern outlived the cause?

When the answer is the third, the approach shifts. The body no longer needs treating. The brain needs teaching. It needs to learn that the war is over, that the signals it is still responding to are echoes, not evidence. That retraining is often the final piece that allows recovery to complete.

The body must feel safe before it can heal. And sometimes, safety is not something you remove a threat to find. It is something you have to rebuild, one nervous system response at a time.

The Mindset Layer

I want to address mindset honestly, because it is real, but it isn't what most people think it is.

Pharmaceutical companies factor in a thirty percent allowance for placebo in drug trials. A third of the therapeutic effect in any intervention comes from the patient's belief that it will work. The mind's influence on the body is measurable, reproducible, and clinically significant.

But here is the distinction this chapter is built on: mindset does not operate independently of the nervous system. Positive thinking, gratitude, visualisation — these practices work best when the nervous system is calm enough to receive them. Telling someone whose body is locked in threat mode to think positively is like telling someone whose house is on fire to enjoy the architecture. The instruction is not wrong. It is badly timed.

The teacher I mentioned earlier, the one whose IBS halved with breath work alone, came back four months later. Her nervous system had shifted, her digestion was stable, and her sleep had normalised. And for the first time in years, she had started a daily meditation practice that actually worked. Her nervous system was finally stable enough for the practice to land. The foundation had changed. So the input finally produced a result.

That is how mindset works in recovery. When the nervous system has shifted, when the body feels safe, when cortisol is settling and digestion is working and sleep is restoring, then mindset practices become powerful. A daily meditation practice, even ten minutes, produces measurable changes in stress hormones, inflammation, and brain function. Gratitude practices shift attention toward recovery rather than threat. These are neurological inputs.

But they belong on a foundation. And the foundation is nervous system regulation. Get the state right first. Then the mindset work lands.

This chapter closes the foundations. Food stabilises the body, sleep repairs it, Movement builds capacity. And the nervous system determines whether any of those inputs can be used. If the system is stuck in threat mode, the best diet, the best sleep hygiene, and the best exercise programme will all underperform. The nervous system is the gatekeeper.

With these foundations in place, or at least understood and actively being addressed, the next stage becomes possible. Because foundations alone are not enough. To move from stabilisation to resolution, you need data. You need to see what is happening inside the body, not guess based on symptoms.

That is where testing begins. And that is where the precision of this approach becomes visible.

A simple breathwork and nervous system regulation guide, including the protocols described in this chapter, is available at TheHealingHierarchy.com.

The foundations are now in place. What comes next requires data, and data changes everything.

PART III

DATA: FIND IT BEFORE YOU FIX IT

Chapter Eight

Why You Need Data (and Why You Don't Need All of It)

Diane had been to four practitioners in two years. A GP, an endocrinologist, a naturopath, and a nutritionist. She had been tested — standard bloods, thyroid panel, full blood count. Every time, the same response: your labs look fine.

She did not feel fine. She was exhausted by mid-afternoon despite sleeping eight hours. Her digestion hadn't been right in over a year. Her mood was flat in a way she could not explain. She was gaining weight despite eating well and exercising regularly. And every practitioner she saw looked at her results, confirmed that everything was within range, and sent her home with the same conclusion: there is nothing clinically wrong.

When she sat in my clinic, I didn't just start with more tests. I started with more precise ones. An advanced functional blood panel, not the standard GP request, this told a different story:"

Vitamin D — 52 nmol/L (21 ng/mL). Lab range starts at 50 nmol/L (20 ng/mL). Optimal starts at 80 nmol/L (32 ng/mL). Technically normal. Functionally inadequate.

B12 — 220 pmol/L (298 pg/mL). Above the deficiency threshold of 200 pmol/L (270 pg/mL). Well below the optimal level of 500 pmol/L (680 pg/mL) where the body performs well.

Fasting insulin — 14 mIU/L. Inside the lab range of less than 20, but above the optimal threshold of less than 10. Early insulin resistance that a standard glucose test would miss entirely.

Ferritin — 33 µg/L. Inside the conventional range, but well below the functional optimal of 50 to 200. Her GP had noted it was on the lower end and prescribed an iron supplement twelve months earlier. It hadn't moved. Nobody had asked why.

Her labs were fine. Her body wasn't.

The Problem with Normal

This is the single most common failure point in conventional medicine for the patients who end up in my clinic. They aren't sick enough to trigger a diagnosis, but they are far enough from optimal function that they feel it in every system. Fatigued. Inflamed. Reactive. Gaining weight. Losing sleep. And being told, repeatedly, that nothing is wrong.

The issue is that laboratory reference ranges are not designed to identify optimal function. They are designed to identify disease. A reference range is calculated from a population average, which means it includes people who are already unwell, sedentary, metabolically compromised, or sub-clinically deficient. Falling within that range means you are statistically normal. It doesn't mean you are functioning well.

Functional ranges are narrower. They represent the levels at which the body performs optimally. Not the levels at which disease has not yet been diagnosed. The gap between the bottom of the lab range and the bottom of the functional range is where many of my patients live. It is the space where symptoms are real, suffering is real, and the standard system has nothing to offer because the numbers do not yet qualify as a diagnosable condition.

Diane lived in that gap for two years. Every test she had was read against laboratory ranges designed to detect disease. Nobody read them against the ranges designed to detect dysfunction. The numbers were the same. The interpretation was completely different.

Your labs fall within the average range, but you don't want average health — which is often unhealthy - you want optimal function.

Symptoms Point. Data Decides.

Symptoms are information. They are the body's way of signalling that something is out of balance. But they are imprecise. A symptom tells you something is wrong. It doesn't tell you what, how much, or why.

Fatigue is the clearest example. A patient presenting with persistent fatigue could be dealing with any of the following: iron deficiency, thyroid dysfunction, mitochondrial underperformance, blood sugar instability, gut dysbiosis, chronic inflammation, poor sleep architecture, adrenal insufficiency, or neurotransmitter depletion. The symptom is the same. The causes are entirely different. The treatment for each one is different. If you guess wrong, you waste time, money, and the patient's trust.

I could have five different patients walk into my clinic with identical IBS symptoms: alternating constipation and diarrhoea, gas, bloating, cramps, reflux, and their stool tests will come back completely different. One has methane-dominant SIBO (small intestinal bacterial overgrowth) driving constipation. Another has a parasitic infection. A third has poor fat metabolism from a sluggish gallbladder. A fourth has severe food intolerances caused by intestinal permeability. The fifth has bacterial dysbiosis with depleted beneficial flora. Same symptoms. Five different treatment plans. Without testing, I am guessing. Guessing in a sensitised system is dangerous, because the wrong intervention can make things worse.

Interpreting symptoms alone is not adequate to understand what is happening on the inside.

Test Strategically, Not Obsessively

If symptoms alone are not enough, the temptation is to test everything. Run every panel. Order every specialty test. Accumulate as much data as possible and then try to make sense of it.

This is a mistake. More testing does not always mean more clarity. It can mean more confusion, more cost, and more anxiety. I have seen patients arrive with folders full of results from a dozen different tests — genetics, mycotoxins, food sensitivity panels, hair mineral analysis, comprehensive hormone profiles, and they are more lost than when they started. They have data. They don't have a plan. The data has not been synthesised into a coherent picture. Nobody has told them which findings matter most, which ones are secondary, and which ones will resolve on their own once the primary imbalances are corrected.

Strategic testing means starting with the tests that give you the broadest, most clinically useful picture of the body's core systems, and then adding specificity only when the initial data points you somewhere. It means testing with a plan, not testing for reassurance.

The difference between a useful test and a wasted one is not the test itself. It is whether someone knows what to do with the result.

A note on what this book can and cannot do.

The chapters that follow will teach you how to read your own data — how to understand what each marker means, how the three tests interact, and how the Healing Hierarchy determines which findings matter most. That understanding is powerful. It will change how you evaluate practitioners, how you ask questions, and how you make decisions about your own health.

But understanding the framework and executing it correctly are different skills. Interpreting a single marker in isolation is simple. Interpreting the pattern across forty markers, where one finding changes the clinical significance of another, where a supplement that is right for one pattern is contraindicated in a different one, and where sequencing errors can set a patient back months — requires pattern recognition built across thousands of cases. The framework scales. The clinical precision required to apply it at the individual level is something that develops with experience, supervision, and feedback.

This book gives you the map. For the foundations, diet, sleep, movement, and nervous system regulation, you have everything you need to begin immediately. For the clinical layers, test interpretation, supplement sequencing, and protocol adjustment, you will need a practitioner. But you will not need them in the same way. You will walk in knowing what to ask, what to test, and what the results should look like. That changes the conversation entirely.

The Essential Trilogy

After thousands of patients and years of clinical practice, I have refined the starting point to three tests. I call them the Essential Trilogy: an advanced blood panel, an advanced stool analysis, and an organic acids test. Between them, they provide a whole-system snapshot that covers the vast majority of what needs to be understood before treatment begins.

The advanced blood panel reveals metabolic health, inflammation, nutrient status, thyroid function, hormone levels, and liver and kidney function. It is the broadest single test available and it should be the baseline for everyone. But, and this is critical, it must be an advanced panel read against functional ranges, not a standard GP panel read against laboratory ranges. The standard panel misses too much, it rarely includes fasting insulin, zinc, copper, or homocysteine. And the markers it does include, like vitamin D and ferritin, are interpreted against ranges wide enough to miss a patient who is functionally depleted.

The advanced stool test (I use a DNA-based stool analysis such as the GI-MAP) reveals what is happening inside the gut. Bacterial balance, parasites, fungal overgrowth, inflammation markers, intestinal permeability, digestive function, detoxification pathways, and immune defence. This is the test I run on every patient, without exception. I am amazed at the number of people I see who have visited multiple practitioners before me and never had an adequate stool test. The gut influences every system in the body — mood, energy, hormones, skin, brain function, immune regulation. If you don't test the gut, you are missing the single most influential system in the recovery process.

The organic acids test is a urine test that reveals what the blood panel and stool test can't see. Mitochondrial function, how well your cells produce energy. Neurotransmitter metabolism, whether serotonin, dopamine, and other brain chemicals are being produced and processed correctly. Detoxification capacity. Methylation function. Systemic yeast, fungal, and bacterial markers that may not appear in the stool because they exist elsewhere in the body. B vitamin status at a cellular level. It often reveals patterns that blood and stool testing cannot capture, which is why I consider it essential.

When I ran all three tests on Diane, the picture changed completely. Her blood panel had already shown the functional deficiencies her previous practitioners had missed. But the stool test revealed a bacterial imbalance and elevated intestinal permeability that explained her digestive symptoms and her inability to absorb the nutrients she was eating. The organic acids test showed early mitochondrial underperformance and depleted methylation markers, which explained the fatigue that no amount of sleep was resolving.

No single test told the full story. Together, they showed a pattern: a gut barrier problem was driving nutrient depletion, which was driving cellular energy failure, which was driving every symptom she had reported to four practitioners over two years. The sequence became clear. The starting point became obvious.

Together, these three tests give you a map. Not a complete map. No single set of tests captures everything. But a map detailed enough to know where to start, what to prioritise, and what sequence to follow. That is what testing is for. Not certainty. Clarity.

THE ESSENTIAL TRILOGY

	BLOOD PANEL	STOOL TEST	ORGANIC ACIDS
WHAT IT MEASURES	Nutrients, thyroid, inflammation, hormones, blood sugar, cholesterol	Gut barrier, infections, microbiome, digestion, beneficial bacteria, H. pylori	Mitochondria, B vitamins, neurotransmitters, detox, bacteria & fungal markers
WHAT IT REVEALS	Deficiencies hiding behind 'normal' ranges	Why the gut is driving symptoms elsewhere	Cellular function that blood tests cannot see
KEY MARKERS	Ferritin, Active B12, homocysteine, CRP, fasting glucose & insulin	Zonulin, calprotectin, secretory IgA, pathogens	MMA, pyroglutamic acid, HVA, VMA, oxalates, Clostridia & yeast markers

Where Testing Goes Wrong

The most consequential testing mistake is running tests without a framework to interpret them. A test result is not a treatment plan. It is a data point. The value is in the synthesis — combining results across all three tests, cross-referencing markers, identifying patterns, and building a sequenced intervention based on what the data reveals together. A single elevated marker in isolation can mean half a dozen things. The same marker in the context of three tests narrows it to one or two. Testing without someone who can synthesise the picture is like getting an MRI with nobody to read it.

This is the error I see most often: patients who have been tested extensively but never had their results integrated into a coherent clinical picture. They have twenty pages of data and no sequence. They start addressing every out-of-range marker at once, which is a guaranteed way to overwhelm a sensitised system. The data isn't the problem. The absence of a plan is the problem.

The second common error is reacting to every result before the foundations are in place. I run the Trilogy early because I want the full picture from day one. But I know that some of what the data shows, particularly cortisol, blood sugar, and inflammation markers, reflects the chaos of a destabilised system. Those markers will shift once sleep, food, and nervous system regulation are addressed. The risk is treating a marker that would have corrected itself, or adding supplements or protocols that target a symptom of instability rather than a true underlying driver. Test early. Act in sequence.

The third is testing too much, too soon. Ordering every available panel at once creates data overload without a framework to interpret it. Start with the Trilogy. Let the data guide what comes next.

And the fourth, the one that surprises most people, is not retesting. You have run the tests, identified the imbalances, started the protocol. How do you know it is working? You retest. It is the mechanism that confirms whether the intervention has produced the intended effect, whether the dose is correct, and whether the body has responded. Without retesting, you are back to guessing, just with more expensive guesses.

A note on cost, because this matters. I do not retest everything every time. Blood work is the most accessible and the most frequently repeated — annually at minimum, and more often for specific markers that are actively being treated. If a stool test has revealed a parasite or pathogen, I will retest that marker specifically, often with a targeted PCR rather than repeating the full panel. For other stool and OAT markers, after hundreds of retests across my patient base, I know which markers reliably clear with specific protocols and which ones need confirmation. In an ideal world, every patient would repeat the full Trilogy annually. A blood panel every year, an OAT or stool test every couple of years once things are running well, and targeted retesting of problem markers in between is realistic. The principle stays the same: test, interpret, intervene, retest, adjust. The frequency adapts to the budget and the clinical picture.

Diane started with the gut. Within eight weeks, her digestion had improved, her energy had begun to return, and her mood had shifted for the first time in two years. We had not tried to treat everything at once. The data showed us where to begin, and we began there.

The next chapter walks through the Essential Trilogy in detail: what each test measures, what it reveals, what it misses, and how the three tests work together to produce a picture that no single test could provide alone. This is where the precision of the approach becomes tangible, where numbers replace assumptions and the body's actual state becomes visible for the first time.

Data does not replace clinical judgment. But it makes clinical judgment possible.

Not sure which tests to start with? A side-by-side comparison of the Essential Trilogy, including what each test reveals, cost ranges, and decision logic, is available at TheHealingHierarchy.com.

Three tests. One picture. That is where precision begins.

Chapter Nine

The Essential Trilogy

Megan had been tired for three years. Not sleepy. Not lazy. Tired in a way that sleep did not fix, that coffee masked for an hour and a half before the fog rolled back in. She was thirty-eight, ate well, exercised three times a week, and had been told by two GPs and a naturopath that her blood work was normal. By the time she sat in my clinic, she had a short list of things she knew were wrong, fatigue, bloating, brain fog, mood crashes in the second half of her cycle, and a longer list of things nobody had been able to explain.

I told her we were going to run three tests. Not a wider set than what she had already done. A more precise one. And I told her something that changed the way she understood the entire process: it was what the three tests revealed together. The patterns that emerged when you laid the results side by side and read them as a system. One test shows you a wall. Three tests show you the building.

Three tests. And what they revealed together finally made sense of everything Megan had been experiencing.

The Advanced Blood Panel

The blood panel is the broadest single test available and the one I order for every patient without exception. It reveals the state of the body's systemic biochemistry — metabolic health, inflammation, nutrient levels, thyroid function, hormone status, and organ function. It is the baseline from which everything else is measured.

But it must be the right panel, read the right way. A standard GP blood test typically includes a full blood count, basic liver function, glucose, and sometimes a thyroid screening — TSH alone. That isn't enough. It misses too many markers that matter, and the ones it does include are read against laboratory reference ranges that, as we discussed, are designed to detect disease rather than dysfunction.

The advanced panel I use includes:

1. B12 and active B12, because total B12 can look adequate while the form the body uses is depleted. Active B12 should be above 80 pmol/L.

2. Vitamin D, which I want to see above 80 nmol/L (32 ng/mL in US units), not merely above the lab threshold of 50 nmol/L (20 ng/mL).

3. A full thyroid panel: TSH (optimal 0.4–2.0 mIU/L), free T3 (optimal 4.0–5.5 pmol/L or 3.0–4.0 pg/mL), free T4 (optimal 14–20 pmol/L or 1.0–1.8 ng/dL), TPO antibodies, and thyroglobulin antibodies, because TSH alone can look normal while the thyroid is under autoimmune attack.

4. Fasting glucose and fasting insulin together, because glucose can remain stable for years while insulin climbs undetected, and by the time glucose rises, the metabolic dysfunction is already well established.

5. Iron studies including ferritin, which I want between 50 and 200 µg/L (same units in both AU and US), not at 33, where you are technically not anaemic but functionally depleted.

6. CRP for systemic inflammation (optimal below 1 mg/L).

7. Homocysteine for methylation and cardiovascular risk.

8. Zinc and copper, because their ratio affects immune function, thyroid health, and neurotransmitter production.

9. MTHFR gene variants (explored in full in Chapter 15), which affect how the body processes folate and drives the methylation cycle.

10. Plus a cholesterol panel read for pattern, not just total number.

That is a substantial panel. But every marker on it earns its place because it reveals something that changes the clinical decision. If B12 is low, the question is why — poor intake, poor absorption, or a gut problem preventing uptake. If thyroid antibodies are elevated, the question is what is driving the immune attack — usually gut permeability. If insulin is climbing while glucose is still normal, the question is how to intervene before full metabolic dysfunction develops. Deficiencies are symptoms. Patterns are systems. The blood panel reveals both.

The panel also includes a reproductive hormone profile, which differs by sex. For both, the starting point is luteinising hormone (LH) and follicle-stimulating hormone (FSH) — pituitary signals that reveal whether the hormonal cascade is being driven correctly from the brain. Low testosterone or irregular cycles can originate in the brain, the adrenals, or the gonads, and the treatment for each is different.

For men: total testosterone, free testosterone, oestradiol, DHEA-S, prolactin, cortisol, and PSA. The key clinical insight is that free testosterone, the biologically active form, can be depleted even when total testosterone looks adequate, particularly when sex hormone binding globulin (SHBG) is elevated. And elevated oestradiol in men, driven by the aromatase enzyme converting testosterone to oestrogen, often explains symptoms attributed to low testosterone alone.

For women: oestradiol, progesterone (tested on Day 21 for accurate luteal-phase reading), LH, FSH, androgens including testosterone and DHEA-S, prolactin, and cortisol. The oestradiol-to-progesterone ratio is often more clinically useful than either value alone — oestrogen dominance relative to progesterone is one of the most common hormonal patterns I see, driving PMS, irregular cycles, mood instability, and difficulty conceiving.

For women who are post-menopausal or peri-menopausal, the picture shifts. Day 21 progesterone is no longer relevant, and LH and FSH are expected to be elevated rather than cyclical. The clinical focus moves to oestradiol decline and its downstream effects on bone density, cardiovascular risk, cognitive function, and tissue integrity. DHEA-S and testosterone remain important — they decline with age and drive the fatigue and loss of resilience that many women are told is simply part of ageing. It is not. It is measurable, and in many cases, addressable. The same upstream principle applies: before considering hormone replacement, assess the gut, inflammation, methylation, and nutrient status. The hormonal picture often improves once those systems are supported.

Chapter 12 walks through the clinical decision framework for hormonal support during this transition, including when bioidentical hormones become appropriate.

One critical point, and this connects directly to the Healing Hierarchy. Hormones are downstream: insulin resistance suppresses SHBG, gut dysbiosis impairs hormone clearance through beta-glucuronidase elevation, chronic inflammation disrupts the hypothalamic-pituitary axis. In my clinical experience, when the gut is repaired, the biochemistry is balanced, and the inflammatory load is reduced, the hormones frequently come back into line without direct treatment. The blood panel captures the hormonal picture. The Trilogy reveals why the hormones are where they are.

Megan's blood panel showed B12 at the low end of the functional range, ferritin at 35 — technically not anaemic, but well below optimal. Her fasting insulin was creeping upward. Her progesterone was low relative to oestradiol, which explained the mood crashes in her luteal phase. And her vitamin D was sitting at 58 nmol/L (23 ng/mL) — inside the lab range, outside the functional one. Any practitioner could have looked at these results and started supplementing. But I wanted to know *why* her nutrients were depleted before I started replacing them. For that, I needed the second test.

What the blood panel misses: it can't see inside the gut. It doesn't measure mitochondrial function. It tells you nothing about detoxification capacity or neurotransmitter metabolism. It can't detect systemic yeast, fungal, or bacterial overgrowth that exists outside the bloodstream. For those, you need the other two tests.

The Advanced Stool Test

If the blood panel shows what is happening in the body's systemic biochemistry, the stool test shows what is happening in the command centre. The gut influences mood, energy, hormones, skin, brain function, and immune regulation. It is the single most influential system in the recovery process. And it is the test I am most often surprised to find patients have never had, even after years of chronic illness and multiple practitioners.

The advanced stool analysis I use is a DNA-based panel such as the GI-MAP. It goes far beyond a standard stool culture. It identifies the full microbial landscape: which bacteria are present and at what levels, whether parasites are present, whether fungal or yeast overgrowth exists. But it also measures a set of functional markers that most practitioners do not request, and these are often the most clinically useful findings on the entire test.

The stool test measures five critical markers:

1. Calprotectin — gut wall inflammation. When elevated, the lining is inflamed, like a wound that won't heal.

2. Pancreatic elastase — digestive enzyme output. When low, food isn't being broken down properly, which means nutrients aren't being absorbed no matter what the patient eats.

3. Secretory IgA — the gut's first line of immune defence. When low, the mucus barrier that protects the intestinal wall is offline and pathogens operate unchecked.

4. Zonulin — intestinal permeability, commonly called leaky gut. When elevated, the tight junctions that regulate what passes through the gut wall have been damaged. Larger molecules, food particles, and bacterial fragments, pass into the bloodstream, triggering the immune system repeatedly. Over time, this creates food intolerances, systemic inflammation, and in some patients, autoimmune disease.

5. Beta-glucuronidase — a detoxification pathway in the gut. When elevated, the body is recirculating toxins and hormones that should have been eliminated.

Then there is the microbial picture itself. Pathogenic bacteria such as Klebsiella, Citrobacter, or H. pylori. Parasites including Blastocystis or Dientamoeba. Fungal overgrowth including Candida species. And equally important — the levels of beneficial bacteria. Low Lactobacillus, low Bifidobacterium, and elevated opportunistic E. coli are patterns I see repeatedly, and they change the treatment approach entirely.

Megan's stool test explained the bloating immediately. Her pancreatic elastase was low. She wasn't producing enough digestive enzymes to break down food properly. Her zonulin was elevated, confirming intestinal permeability. Her beneficial bacteria were depleted, with low Lactobacillus and low Bifidobacterium, and she had elevated beta-glucuronidase, meaning her gut was recirculating oestrogen instead of eliminating it, which was compounding the hormonal imbalance her blood panel had already flagged. The bloating was not a food sensitivity. It was a digestive capacity problem sitting on top of a gut barrier problem. And the hormonal picture was not separate from the gut picture. The gut *was* the hormonal picture.

What the stool test misses: it can't measure systemic inflammation outside the gut. It tells you nothing about nutrient levels in the blood, mitochondrial function, or neurotransmitter metabolism. It doesn't capture microbial overgrowth that exists outside the gastrointestinal tract, in the sinuses, the urinary tract, or systemically. For that, you need the third test.

The Organic Acids Test

The organic acids test is a urine test that measures over seventy metabolite markers — small byproducts of the body's cellular activity. It is a comprehensive assessment that reveals what is happening at the biochemical level, inside the cells and pathways that the blood panel and stool test can't see. In my clinical experience, it is the test that most reliably reveals hidden drivers that explain why patients are not improving despite doing everything else correctly.

The test measures several critical domains.

1. First, yeast and fungal markers, including Candida and Aspergillus indicators. These are markers of systemic fungal overgrowth that may not appear on a stool test because the overgrowth exists outside the gut, in other areas of the body. When these markers are elevated, the patient is often dealing with fatigue, brain fog, and immune dysfunction that won't resolve until the fungal burden is addressed.

2. Second, Clostridia bacterial markers. Clostridia species can inhibit the production of neurotransmitters in the brain — contributing to depression, anxiety, sleep disturbance, and mood instability. This is one of the most clinically significant findings on the OAT, because it reveals a direct biochemical mechanism behind symptoms that are often dismissed as psychological.

3. Third, the Krebs cycle and mitochondrial markers. The mitochondria are the energy-producing structures inside most cells. They generate ATP — adenosine triphosphate, which is the body's primary energy molecule. When Krebs cycle markers such as succinic acid, fumaric acid, malic acid, or citric acid are elevated, it indicates that energy production is impaired. The patient feels exhausted not because they need more sleep or more willpower, but because their cells are not generating energy efficiently. The causes can include B vitamin deficiency, CoQ10 depletion, toxic exposure, or ongoing microbial burden. This is the test that turns fatigue from a vague complaint into a measurable dysfunction.

4. Fourth, neurotransmitter metabolites. The OAT measures markers related to serotonin, dopamine, and other brain chemicals. Not the neurotransmitters themselves, but the metabolic byproducts that indicate whether production and processing pathways are functioning correctly. Low serotonin metabolites in a patient with depression and poor sleep expand the clinical picture significantly. They suggest that cofactor support and gut health may need to be addressed alongside any existing treatment, and they give the practitioner a measurable pathway to track rather than relying on symptom reporting alone.

5. Fifth, methylation and detoxification markers. Glutathione, the body's master antioxidant, can be assessed through pyroglutamic acid. B vitamin status at a cellular level, including B2, B6, and B12 through methylmalonic acid. These markers reveal whether the body's detoxification and repair pathways are functioning or bottlenecked.

6. And sixth, oxalate metabolites. Elevated oxalates are often driven by underlying yeast or fungal overgrowth, not excessive oxalate consumption. They can contribute to kidney stones, joint pain, neurological symptoms, and chronic inflammation. Clearing the underlying microbial driver usually resolves the oxalate problem — restricting oxalate-rich foods is a temporary measure, not a solution.

Megan's OAT was the test that explained the fatigue. Her Krebs cycle markers were elevated across three of the six intermediaries, succinic acid, fumaric acid, and 2-oxoglutaric acid, indicating that her mitochondria were not producing energy efficiently. Her pyroglutamic acid was elevated, signalling depleted glutathione and a detoxification bottleneck. And her serotonin metabolites were on the low side, which correlated with the mood crashes her blood panel had already hinted at through the progesterone-oestradiol imbalance. The fatigue was not in her head. It was in her mitochondria. The mood instability was not purely hormonal. It had a biochemical production pathway that could be measured and addressed.

The OAT is the test that most often explains what everything else could not. But its real power only becomes visible when the results sit alongside the other two.

How the Three Tests Work Together

No single test tells the full story. The power of the Trilogy is not in any one result — it is in the cross-referencing. When the blood panel, stool test, and OAT are interpreted together, patterns emerge that no single test could reveal on its own. Without integration, data is noise. With sequence, data becomes direction.

This is what happened with Megan. Each test in isolation told a partial story. The blood panel showed nutrient depletion and a hormonal imbalance. A practitioner working from that alone might have supplemented B12, iron, and vitamin D, added progesterone support, and called it a plan. The stool test showed impaired digestion, a compromised gut barrier, and disrupted oestrogen elimination. A practitioner working from that alone might have started gut repair and antimicrobials. The OAT showed mitochondrial underperformance, depleted glutathione, and low serotonin metabolites. A practitioner working from that alone might have started mitochondrial cofactors and mood support.

But laid together, the three tests told one story.

Megan's gut barrier was compromised, which was impairing nutrient absorption, which explained the low B12 and ferritin despite a good diet. Providing more of these would provide limited improvement if she could not absorb them.

The impaired absorption was starving her mitochondria of the cofactors they needed to produce energy, which explained the fatigue. The elevated beta-glucuronidase was recirculating oestrogen, which explained the hormonal imbalance and the mood crashes. The depleted glutathione was bottlenecking her detoxification, which meant her body couldn't clear the inflammatory load the leaky gut was generating.

The sequence became clear. Gut first: repair the barrier, restore digestive capacity, rebalance the microbiome. Then nutrient repletion: once absorption was functioning, the supplements would reach the cells that needed them. Then mitochondrial and detox support: once the upstream problems were resolved, the energy and detoxification systems could be rebuilt on a stable foundation. The hormones, I suspected, would begin to correct on their own once the gut was no longer recirculating oestrogen and the inflammatory load had dropped.

Three tests. One integrated picture. One clear starting point.

This is what I mean by decision architecture. The individual results are data. The pattern across all three tests is the diagnosis. The diagnosis determines the sequence. Without all three layers, you are making decisions with partial information, and partial information in a sensitised system leads to partial results at best and setbacks at worst.

When to Go Further

The Trilogy is the starting point. It isn't always the end point. Depending on what the initial data reveals, additional investigations may be warranted. A SIBO breath test if the stool test and symptoms suggest small intestinal bacterial overgrowth. Mycotoxin testing if the organic acids test shows markers consistent with mould exposure. Genetic testing, particularly MTHFR and other methylation variants, if the blood panel and OAT suggest methylation dysfunction that warrants deeper investigation. Hair mineral tissue analysis if heavy metal burden is suspected. A comprehensive hormone panel if the blood results flag thyroid, adrenal, or sex hormone irregularities that need further detail.

But these are second-line tests. They are guided by the Trilogy, not ordered alongside it. Running a mycotoxin panel on a patient who has never had a stool test is like checking the wiring in a house before confirming the foundation is sound. It might find something. But it is out of sequence. And out of sequence means out of context, which means the result is harder to interpret and easier to misapply.

Reading the Picture

Once the data is in, the clinical question becomes: where do you start? The Healing Hierarchy provides the framework, but the data provides the specifics. In practice, this means clustering the findings into system patterns and identifying which system is generating the most downstream disruption.

Symptoms and markers tend to cluster.

Bloating, constipation or diarrhoea, food reactions, skin issues, and autoimmune flares point to the gut system, and the stool test will usually confirm it.

Fatigue, brain fog, poor recovery, and exercise intolerance point to energy and mitochondrial function, and the OAT will clarify.

PMS, irregular cycles, low libido, thyroid symptoms, and testosterone drift point to hormonal dysfunction, and the blood panel will show whether the driver is thyroid, metabolic, or nutrient-based.

Chemical sensitivity, histamine reactions, and poor tolerance of supplements point to a detox bottleneck, and the OAT's glutathione and methylation markers will confirm.

Frequent infections, slow wound healing, and chronic inflammation point to immune dysregulation. Secretory IgA, CRP, and calprotectin across the stool and blood tests will show the state of the immune system.

The clinical method is simple in principle, demanding in execution: measure, decide, act, retest.

- Measure - gather the data through the Trilogy.
- Decide - identify the priority system based on the Healing Hierarchy and the pattern the data reveals.
- Act - intervene on the priority system first, using a sequenced protocol.
- Retest - confirm the intervention worked, adjust if it didn't, and move to the next system.

This cycle repeats. It is not a one-time event. It is the operating logic of the entire recovery process.

Tracking symptoms alongside this process matters, not obsessively, but consistently. The objective data from the Trilogy tells you what is happening inside the body. The subjective data from symptom tracking tells you how the body is responding to what you are doing about it. Together, they create a feedback loop that makes each decision more precise than the last.

In practice, this means tracking weekly rather than daily. Daily tracking tends to amplify noise. A bad night of sleep, a stressful day at work, a meal that didn't sit well. Weekly tracking smooths the noise into patterns. Rate each system on a simple severity scale: energy, digestion, mood, sleep, pain, mental clarity. Note what improved, what stayed the same, what worsened. Note any obvious triggers — a food reintroduction, a supplement change, a period of high stress, travel. The goal is not to catalogue every fluctuation. It is to identify trends over four to eight weeks that either confirm the protocol is working or signal that something needs adjusting.

A bad week is not a crisis. Two bad weeks in a row is not necessarily a crisis either. It may be a healing response as the body clears pathogens or adjusts to a new supplement. But three or four weeks of worsening in a specific system, despite following the protocol, is data. It tells you either the intervention is not addressing the right driver, the dose needs adjusting, or a new variable has entered the picture. That is when you reassess. It may mean adjusting the dose, changing the intervention, or in some cases, retesting a specific marker. Symptom tracking is what keeps you honest between tests — it is the early warning system that prevents months of drift before the next round of data confirms what you could have caught at week three.

The Trilogy gives you a whole-system snapshot. It maps three biological layers: systemic function, microbial terrain, and cellular metabolism, and shows how they interact. It is the foundation of every treatment plan I build, and it is the reason patients who have seen multiple practitioners without progress begin to see change within weeks of starting a properly sequenced protocol.

Megan started with the gut. We repaired her intestinal barrier, restored digestive enzyme output, and rebalanced her microbiome over twelve weeks. When we retested, her zonulin had normalised, her elastase had improved, and her beta-glucuronidase had dropped. Her bloating was gone. We then moved to nutrient repletion, and this time, with the gut functioning properly, her B12 and ferritin climbed steadily. By month four her energy had shifted, and by month five her mood crashes had softened. We never treated her hormones. We treated the reason they were misbehaving. When the gut stopped recirculating oestrogen and the nutrient supply to her mitochondria was restored, the downstream systems corrected on their own. When upstream systems stabilise, downstream systems often correct without force. That is what sequenced recovery looks like when it is driven by data rather than guesswork.

It is also, for most readers of this book, the moment where this stops being theory and becomes personal. You can read about the Healing Hierarchy and understand it intellectually. But when you see your own numbers — your own zonulin level, your own mitochondrial markers, your own B12 and insulin and thyroid antibodies — the picture stops being abstract. It becomes yours. And that is when the work begins.

Understanding these markers is the first step. Knowing which ones are driving your specific pattern, and in what order to address them, is the clinical skill that turns data into a recovery plan. The chapters ahead show you exactly how that process works, system by system.

The next four chapters walk through the major systems one by one, gut, energy, hormones, and mood, each anchored by a patient case study that shows how the Trilogy data drove the clinical decisions and what happened when the sequence was followed correctly.

The testing options, interpretation guides, and symptom tracking tools referenced in this chapter are available at TheHealingHierarchy.com. If you want to see your own data through the lens this chapter teaches, that is where the Essential Trilogy, the interpretation framework, and the optimal ranges all come together.

The chapters ahead — gut, energy, hormones, mood, genetics, environment — each have a scoring exercise in the companion workbook that maps your clinical picture against the patterns in this book. Without the workbook, you will read the cases and think "that sounds like me." With the workbook, you will know.

TheHealingHierarchy.com/workbook

PART IV
SYSTEMS RESTORATION

Chapter Ten

The Gut: Health Begins Here

By the time Sarah reached her late fifties, she had stopped expecting to feel well. For more than a decade, she had lived with the understanding that her immune system was attacking itself. A diagnosis that explained her joint pain, skin flares, fatigue, and digestive issues, but offered little hope of resolution. Each flare reinforced the same message: this was something to manage, not reverse.

She was exhausted by it. She had tried multiple diets, supplements, medications, and alternative therapies. Each offered short-term improvement followed by relapse. She had learned to live around her symptoms, but she never felt well. And then a severe COVID infection pushed her body past a point it couldn't recover from on its own. After that, every food seemed to trigger inflammation, her joint pain worsened, and her energy collapsed further. Her immune system had lost the ability to distinguish friend from foe.

When she sat in my clinic, I didn't start by looking at her immune system. I started by looking at her gut.

Why the Gut Comes First

Every chapter in this book has built toward this point. Earlier chapters established the order through the Healing Hierarchy, stabilised the system through foundations, and provided the data through the Essential Trilogy. Now the question is: where do you start the actual work of restoration? For the majority of patients I see, and I estimate it at eighty per cent or higher, the answer is the gut.

That is not a philosophical preference. It is a clinical observation backed by decades of research and confirmed every week in my practice. The gut is the single most influential system in the body. Approximately seventy to eighty per cent of the immune system is housed in the gut-associated lymphoid tissue. The gut produces or mediates the production of key neurotransmitters — approximately ninety-five per cent of the body's serotonin is produced in the gastrointestinal tract. The gut regulates systemic inflammation through the integrity of the intestinal barrier and the composition of the microbiome. It controls nutrient absorption, which feeds every other system in the body. It influences hormone metabolism through detoxification pathways. And it communicates directly with the brain through the vagus nerve, forming what is known as the gut-brain axis. A bidirectional communication system that means what happens in the gut doesn't stay in the gut.

The research establishing these connections is not emerging. It is settled. The gut microbiome has established communication axes to the liver, the skin, the brain, the kidneys, the lungs, the bones, and the immune system. Alterations in the gut microbiome have been linked to autoimmune disease, metabolic syndrome, mood disorders, skin conditions, neurological dysfunction, and chronic fatigue. This is the biological reality that most conventional treatment still ignores.

In my clinical experience, the gut is the system that most reliably explains why other interventions have not worked. I have seen mood improve, hormones rebalance, skin clear, energy return, and autoimmune markers drop — all from treating the gut alone, without directly touching those other systems. Sometimes I don't even have data on those systems yet. I treat the gut, stabilise the diet, and the downstream improvements begin before I have had time to address anything else. When the gatekeeper is broken, everything downstream fails. Fix the gatekeeper, and the downstream systems often begin to self-correct.

What Goes Wrong

A healthy gut performs three critical functions simultaneously. It digests and absorbs nutrients from food. It maintains a selective barrier, the intestinal wall, that allows nutrients through into the bloodstream while keeping pathogens, toxins, and undigested food particles out. It houses a complex ecosystem of microorganisms. The microbiome. That influences immune regulation, neurotransmitter production, hormone metabolism, and detoxification. When any of these three functions breaks down, the consequences extend far beyond the digestive system.

Intestinal permeability — commonly called leaky gut - is the condition I see most frequently at the root of chronic illness. The intestinal wall is lined with cells held together by tight junctions, which act as gates. In a healthy gut, these gates open selectively to allow nutrients through while keeping everything else out. When the tight junctions are damaged by chronic stress, poor diet, infections, medications such as NSAIDs and antibiotics, alcohol, or environmental toxins — the gates open indiscriminately. Undigested food particles, bacterial fragments, and toxins pass through the intestinal wall into the bloodstream. The immune system recognises these substances as foreign invaders and mounts an inflammatory response. If this happens once, it resolves. If it happens chronically because the barrier remains damaged, the immune system stays in a state of constant activation. Over time, this chronic immune activation drives food intolerances, systemic inflammation, skin conditions, brain fog, joint pain, and, in susceptible individuals, autoimmune disease.

Dysbiosis is the second major pattern. The gut microbiome in a healthy person contains a diverse population of beneficial bacteria, Lactobacillus, Bifidobacterium, and hundreds of other species that keep the ecosystem in balance. When beneficial populations decline and opportunistic or pathogenic organisms take over, the system shifts. Pathogenic bacteria such as Klebsiella, Citrobacter, or H. pylori produce inflammatory toxins. Parasites such as Blastocystis or Dientamoeba disrupt the mucosal lining. Candida and other fungal species overgrow when bacterial competition is removed, often after antibiotic use. Certain bacteria, particularly Clostridia species, can directly interfere with neurotransmitter production, driving mood disturbance, sleep disruption, and anxiety through a purely biochemical mechanism.

The third pattern is impaired digestion. If the body isn't producing enough stomach acid, bile, or digestive enzymes, food is not broken down properly. Undigested food ferments in the gut, producing gas, bloating, and discomfort. Nutrients that should be absorbed are not. The undigested particles irritate the gut lining, contributing to the permeability problem. This is why I see patients who eat well but still show nutrient deficiencies on their blood panel. The issue isn't what they are eating but whether they are digesting and absorbing it.

These three problems reinforce each other. The system needs to be addressed in sequence.

Sarah's Data

Sarah's stool test confirmed everything her symptoms had been signalling for a decade. Her zonulin was 185 ng/mL, normal is below 107. Her intestinal barrier was wide open, letting undigested food and bacterial fragments leak into her bloodstream and trigger immune confusion on a daily basis. Her calprotectin was 285 µg/g — normal is below 50. Her gut lining was chronically inflamed, five times the healthy threshold, like a wound that wouldn't heal.

Her microbial picture was equally clear. Klebsiella and Citrobacter, two opportunistic bacteria known for producing inflammatory toxins, had colonised her gut at severe overgrowth levels. Her beneficial bacteria were depleted. And her secretory IgA was 142 µg/g, against an optimal range of 510 to 2,040. Her gut's immune defence system was nearly offline — unable to keep the pathogens in check, unable to mount the mucosal protection that a healthy gut provides.

Her blood panel added the systemic picture. CRP, the marker for body-wide inflammation, was 8.2 mg/L, against an optimal of below 1.0. Her immune system was on high alert, attacking everything, including her own tissues. That was the autoimmune pattern her previous practitioners had been trying to suppress with medication. But the immune system was not malfunctioning. It was responding appropriately to chronic gut irritation. The inflammation was not the disease. It was the symptom. The gut was the disease.

This is the reframe that changed everything for Sarah. Her immune system was not overactive. It was doing exactly what it was designed to do — responding to a genuine biological threat. The threat was not an external pathogen that had invaded and left. It was an internal environment that had been sending distress signals every day for over a decade. Suppress the immune response without fixing the gut, and you suppress the alarm without putting out the fire.

The Gut Repair Sequence

Gut restoration is not a single intervention. It is a sequenced protocol with five phases, and the order of those phases matters as much as the interventions themselves. Getting the order wrong does not just slow progress. It can actively set the patient back.

The first phase is motility. Getting the system to move spontaneously. Before anything else, waste needs to be moving out of the body. If a patient is constipated, not passing a well-formed stool at least once daily, nothing else will work properly. Toxins that should be eliminated are reabsorbed. Die-off from antimicrobial treatment has nowhere to go. The gut environment becomes stagnant, and stagnation breeds further dysbiosis. Motility support is not glamorous, but it is non-negotiable.

Magnesium, adequate hydration, fibre from whole food sources, and in some cases targeted motility support are the starting points. If the drains are blocked, you don't start running water.

The second phase is digestive support. Once motility is established, the focus shifts to ensuring the body can break down and absorb food. This means assessing and supporting stomach acid production, bile flow from the liver and gallbladder, and pancreatic enzyme output. Low stomach acid, which is far more common than excess acid, particularly in patients over forty, means proteins are not being broken down, minerals are not being absorbed, and partially digested food sits in the stomach and ferments. If bile production is sluggish, fats are not emulsified properly, which means fat-soluble vitamins (A, D, E, K) are not absorbed and the small intestine is not being swept clean — bile acts as a natural antimicrobial that helps prevent bacterial overgrowth in the small intestine. This is why SIBO so often recurs after treatment: the antimicrobials clear the overgrowth, but if bile flow is not restored, the conditions that allowed the overgrowth return. Digestive enzymes, bile salts, and in appropriate cases betaine HCl to support stomach acid are the tools here.

The third phase is gut lining repair. Once motility is working and digestion is supported, the intestinal barrier itself needs to be rebuilt. This is the phase that directly addresses intestinal permeability — sealing the tight junctions that have been damaged. L-glutamine is the primary amino acid used for gut lining repair. It is the preferred fuel source for the cells that line the intestinal wall. Zinc carnosine supports mucosal integrity and has specific anti-inflammatory effects on the gut lining. Collagen and bone broth provide the amino acid building blocks for tissue repair. This phase is critical and must come before aggressive antimicrobial treatment. If you start killing pathogens before the gut lining has begun to repair, the inflammatory debris from the die-off passes through the still-permeable barrier and triggers a systemic immune response. The patient feels worse, not better. Repair before eradication. Always.

The fourth phase is pathogen eradication. Only once motility is established, digestion is supported, and the gut lining repair is underway do I begin targeted antimicrobial treatment. The specific formulations depend on what the stool test has revealed. Bacterial overgrowth, parasitic infection, fungal dominance, and methane-producing organisms each require different antimicrobial strategies. I use targeted herbal blends rather than a single-agent approach, because sensitised patients need precision, not broad-spectrum guessing. Specific spore-based or saccharomyces-based probiotics are used alongside the antimicrobials to support microbial rebalancing, but traditional multi-strain probiotics are generally held until the clearing phase is complete. The goal is not to sterilise the gut. It is to shift the balance, reduce the pathogenic load and create space for beneficial organisms to recolonize

The fifth phase is microbiome rebuilding. After the pathogens have been cleared, the focus shifts to reintroducing microbial diversity. Multi-strain probiotics, fermented foods, and prebiotic fibre that feeds the beneficial bacteria are the tools. This is also the phase where dietary reintroduction can begin carefully — testing which foods the body can now tolerate that it couldn't before, because the immune reactivity that was driving the food intolerances was a consequence of the leaky gut, not a permanent feature of the patient's biology.

Why the Order Matters

Every phase in this sequence exists because of the phase before it. Skip motility and the die-off products have nowhere to go. Start eradication before repair and the inflammatory debris passes through the still-permeable barrier, as described above, the patient gets worse, not better. Add probiotics before clearing pathogens and the beneficial bacteria cannot colonise because the pathogenic organisms are still occupying the terrain. Rebuild the microbiome before fixing digestion and the new bacteria starve because the environment cannot support them.

I have seen every one of these mistakes in patients who arrive in my clinic after previous treatments have failed. The interventions were not wrong. The order was. A practitioner prescribed antimicrobials to clear a bacterial overgrowth, but the patient was constipated and had no motility support. The die-off recirculated, the patient crashed, and the overgrowth returned within months. Another prescribed probiotics and gut-healing supplements, but the patient had active parasites that were never identified — the probiotics could not establish because the parasites were still disrupting the ecosystem. Another put the patient on a gut-repair protocol but never assessed stomach acid or bile flow — the patient continued to absorb nutrients poorly, the gut lining couldn't rebuild without adequate raw materials, and progress stalled.

The Healing Hierarchy applies within gut treatment, not just between systems. The sequence within the gut is as important as the sequence across the body. This is why I treat the gut as a five-phase protocol, not a single-step intervention. Each phase creates the conditions for the next to work.

What Happened with Sarah

Sarah's protocol followed the five phases exactly. Motility and digestive support first. Then four weeks of gut lining repair before we introduced herbal antimicrobials to address the Klebsiella and Citrobacter overgrowth, alongside high-dose probiotics to shift the microbial balance. A Whole Food Reset ran concurrently — gluten, dairy, processed foods, and refined sugars removed, replaced with nutrient-dense whole foods. After eight weeks, slow reintroduction identified gluten and dairy as her primary inflammatory triggers. They were removed long-term.

We supported her methylation and detoxification pathways alongside the gut work, and focused on nervous system regulation because chronic inflammation and a decade of health anxiety had left her stress response in permanent activation. The gut repair would have been slower and less durable without addressing the stress load that was contributing to the permeability in the first place.

At six months, we retested.

Zonulin had dropped from 185 to 68. Normal. Her intestinal barrier was intact for the first time in years. Calprotectin had dropped from 285 to 22 — the chronic gut inflammation was gone and Klebsiella and Citrobacter were back to safe levels. Secretory IgA had risen from 142 to 890, her gut's immune defence was back online and functioning. And CRP, the systemic inflammation marker that had been running at 8.2, was now 0.6. Optimal.

Sarah's autoimmune flares stopped. Her joint pain, which had been constant for years, faded and then disappeared. Her skin cleared. Her digestion became predictable and comfortable for the first time in a decade. Her energy returned steadily. Not the adrenaline-driven good days she used to have, but real, sustainable energy. She described having more energy than she had experienced in years, not just physically but mentally and emotionally.

Perhaps the most meaningful shift was psychological. She no longer felt like she was walking on eggshells around her health — waiting for the next flare, the next reaction, the next setback. Her body felt calm, resilient, and reliable again. For the first time in years, she trusted it. This was stability. The only thing she had got wrong was believing it would never come.

We never suppressed her immune system. We fixed the reason it was activated. Autoimmunity was the label. The gut was the driver. We didn't quiet the alarm. We removed the smoke. And when the gut was repaired, the immune system no longer had a reason to attack.

This is what gut restoration looks like when it is done in sequence, driven by data, and guided by the Healing Hierarchy. It is neither fast nor simple. But it is reliable, because it addresses the system that sits upstream of almost everything else. Fix the gatekeeper, and the downstream systems follow.

Sarah's case followed a clear sequence, but the sequence was not obvious from the data alone. The decision to prioritise barrier repair before antimicrobials, to delay immune modulation until the gut environment could sustain it, and to hold off on nutrient repletion until absorption was functioning — these were clinical judgments informed by thousands of similar cases. The framework gives you the logic. Your own data will give you the specifics. And the distance between the two is where working with someone trained in this methodology makes the difference between a protocol that partially helps and one that resolves the picture.

If you have been told your condition is autoimmune or inflammatory or stress-related or idiopathic, meaning they don't know why, the question worth asking is whether anyone has looked at the gut properly. Not a standard stool culture. A comprehensive, DNA-based stool analysis that measures the functional markers, the microbial landscape, and the integrity of the barrier. Because in my experience, the gut is the answer more often than any other single system. Not always. But more often than most patients or practitioners expect.

The next chapter turns to the second system in the restoration sequence: energy and biochemistry. A different patient. A different pattern. The same principle. That data reveals what is wrong, and sequence determines what to fix first.

SARAH — Autoimmune & Gut Restoration (6 months)

MARKER	BEFORE		AFTER
Zonulin	185 ng/mL	→	68 ng/mL
Calprotectin	285 µg/g	→	22 µg/g
CRP	8.2 mg/L	→	0.6 mg/L
Secretory IgA	142 µg/g	→	890 µg/g
Klebsiella / Citrobacter	Severe overgrowth	→	Cleared

Autoimmune flares stopped. Energy returned. Digestion predictable.

The gut was the gatekeeper. Once it was repaired, everything downstream began to self-correct.

The same Gut Health Pattern Map from the workbook scores your symptoms against the patterns in this chapter. Sarah scored 32 out of 40 before treatment. Three months later, her score was 11. Your turn.

Chapter Eleven

Fatigue Is a Production Problem

James looked like someone who was coping. He ran a business, trained regularly, and pushed through each day on discipline alone. From the outside, he appeared successful and driven. On the inside, his energy was collapsing. Rest did not restore him. Motivation did not translate into stamina. And every good day came at the cost of the next.

He was forty-two. He had a young family, a demanding business, and a body that had stopped keeping up three years earlier. The decline had been gradual at first. A slow erosion of recovery, a creeping brain fog, a flatness in his mood that he couldn't explain. He compensated with caffeine and discipline. Then came the final straw: a severe root canal infection that required emergency treatment. Within months of that infection, his energy collapsed entirely, his concentration fractured, and his motivation disappeared. His body had crossed a line it couldn't come back from on its own.

He had been told, repeatedly, that he was burnt out and needed to slow down. He tried. It didn't help. Every small improvement was followed by a crash. He took time off work, reduced training, cleaned up his diet, tried adrenal and energy supplements. Nothing stuck. Because the problem was not burnout. It was not stress. It was not motivation. It was how his body was producing energy at a cellular level, and something upstream had broken the machinery.

Fatigue Is a Production Problem

The previous chapter established the gut as the first system to address in the restoration sequence. For most patients, that is where the clinical work begins. But the gut isn't the only upstream driver. For a significant number of patients, particularly those presenting with persistent fatigue, brain fog, poor recovery, and mood disturbance that doesn't resolve with gut repair alone.

The second layer is energy production and biochemistry.

Fatigue is a production problem, not motivation, not mindset. Rest does not fix an energy system that can't produce energy. Every cell in the body requires adenosine triphosphate (ATP) to function. ATP is the molecule that powers muscle contraction, nerve signalling, hormone production, immune function, detoxification, and cognitive processing. When ATP production is compromised, every system in the body slows down. The person is not lazy or unmotivated. The cells themselves do not have enough fuel to perform their basic functions.

ATP is produced primarily in the mitochondria. The energy-producing structures inside nearly every cell. The mitochondria run on a metabolic cycle called the Krebs cycle, which converts nutrients into usable energy. That cycle requires specific inputs to function: B vitamins, CoQ10, magnesium, iron, carnitine, stable blood sugar, and adequate oxygen delivery. When any of these inputs is missing or depleted, the cycle slows. Energy output drops. The patient feels it as fatigue. Not the tiredness that follows a long day, but the deep, systemic exhaustion that sleep does not fix.

This is why the label "adrenal fatigue" is misleading. The concept suggests that the adrenal glands are exhausted from chronic stress and have stopped producing cortisol. In most cases, that isn't what is happening. What is happening is mitochondrial underperformance, methylation dysfunction, gut-driven inflammation, or nutrient depletion — sometimes all four at once. The adrenals may be involved, but they are rarely the primary driver. Treating the adrenals without addressing the mitochondria, the methylation pathways, or the gut interference is like changing the oil in a car with a cracked engine block. The oil was not the problem.

Where Energy Breaks Down

In my clinical experience, persistent fatigue traces back to one or more of six common bottlenecks. Each one disrupts the energy production chain at a different point, and each one requires a different intervention. Generic energy supplements rarely work for the same reason. They are guessing at which bottleneck is present without testing to confirm.

The first is nutrient depletion. The Krebs cycle and mitochondrial electron transport chain are enzyme-driven processes that require specific cofactors to operate. B vitamins, particularly B1, B2, B3, B5, B6, and B12, are required at multiple steps. CoQ10 is essential for electron transport. Magnesium is a cofactor in over three hundred enzymatic reactions, including ATP synthesis itself. Iron carries oxygen to the mitochondria. Carnitine transports fatty acids into the mitochondria for fuel. When any of these is depleted - and in chronically ill patients, multiple depletions are common - the energy production line slows or stalls. The organic acids test reveals this directly through Krebs cycle markers; when succinic acid, fumaric acid, or malic acid are elevated, the cycle is struggling at specific enzymatic steps.

The second is methylation dysfunction. Methylation is a biochemical process that occurs billions of times per second in the body, transferring methyl groups from one molecule to another. It is essential for producing neurotransmitters, repairing DNA, building immune cells, processing hormones, and detoxifying chemicals. When methylation is impaired, through genetic variants such as MTHFR, nutrient depletion, or chronic stress, the downstream effects are broad: poor neurotransmitter production, impaired detoxification, elevated homocysteine (a cardiovascular and neurological risk marker), and compromised cellular repair. The patient feels this as fatigue, brain fog, mood instability, and poor stress tolerance. Homocysteine on the blood panel is the primary screening marker. Optimal is between 5 and 7 µmol/L. Below 5 can signal excessive methylation support or high detoxification demand that the body is struggling to sustain. Above 10 warrants investigation. Above 14, as in James's case, indicates significant methylation impairment.

The third is gut-driven biochemical interference. This is the direct link between the previous chapter and this one. Certain pathogenic bacteria, particularly Clostridia species, produce metabolites that directly interfere with neurotransmitter production and energy pathways. Clostridia metabolites such as HPHPA and 4-cresol are measurable on the organic acids test. When elevated, they indicate that a gut infection is actively disrupting the brain's chemical signalling. This is a measurable, testable, treatable pathway. A patient with elevated Clostridia markers will often present with disrupted sleep, low motivation, brain fog, and mood disturbance — all of which resolve when the Clostridia is cleared and the neurotransmitter pathways are supported. This was the pattern James's OAT would reveal.

The fourth is glutathione depletion. Glutathione is the body's master antioxidant. The primary defence against oxidative stress, the key player in detoxification, and a protector of mitochondrial function. When glutathione is depleted, through chronic stress, infection, environmental toxin exposure, or prolonged inflammation — the mitochondria become vulnerable to damage, detoxification slows, and the body accumulates metabolic debris that further impairs energy production. Aconitic acid on the organic acids test is a marker for glutathione status. When it is low, glutathione reserves are depleted. Pyroglutamic acid, when elevated, confirms the depletion from a different angle — the body is burning through glutathione faster than it can replenish.

The fifth is blood sugar instability. The mitochondria need a steady fuel supply. When blood sugar is volatile, spiking after high-carbohydrate meals, then crashing two hours later, the energy production system lurches between overload and starvation. Insulin resistance compounds the problem: cells become less responsive to insulin, glucose cannot enter the cells efficiently, and the mitochondria are starved even when blood sugar is technically elevated. The patient experiences this as energy crashes after meals, afternoon fatigue, sugar cravings, irritability, and poor concentration — all of which are frequently misattributed to stress or poor sleep. Fasting insulin and fasting glucose on the blood panel are the primary screening markers. When fasting insulin is elevated above optimal, even if glucose appears normal, the body is already compensating, and the mitochondrial fuel supply is under strain.

The sixth is chronic inflammation. Inflammation is metabolically expensive. When the immune system is chronically activated, whether from gut permeability, food intolerances, hidden infections, or autoimmune processes, it diverts enormous resources away from energy production and toward immune defence. The body prioritises survival over performance. The result is fatigue that doesn't respond to rest, because the energy is not being lost to activity. It is being consumed by an invisible fire.

James's Data

James's organic acids test was the test that cracked the case. His Krebs cycle markers showed inefficiency at multiple steps. The energy production pathway was underperforming. But the OAT went further. His aconitic acid was low, indicating glutathione depletion. His cellular defence system was running on empty. His pyroglutamic acid was elevated at 38.5, against a normal ceiling of 28, confirming the depletion of glutathione from the high demand: his body was burning through glutathione faster than it could produce it. His vitamin B6 was low. His Clostridia markers, HPHPA and 4-cresol, were significantly elevated. Harmful gut bacteria were producing neurotoxins that were actively disrupting his ability to produce dopamine and other neurotransmitters.

His dopamine precursor marker, homovanillic acid, or HVA, was low. His brain's motivation and drive molecule was running on empty. This was not a psychological problem. It was a biochemical one, driven by a gut infection interfering with a neurotransmitter production pathway.

His blood panel added the hormonal picture. Total testosterone was 265 ng/dL, against an optimal range of 450 to 900. His testosterone had not declined because of ageing. It had collapsed because the upstream systems that support testosterone production, methylation, detoxification, nutrient status, gut health, were all compromised. Homocysteine was 14.8 µmol/L, against an optimal of 5 to 7. His methylation pathway was significantly impaired, which meant his body couldn't efficiently produce neurotransmitters, clear toxins, or support hormonal function.

Three years of sixty-hour work weeks, newborn twins, chronic sleep deprivation, and then the root canal infection. His body had crossed the sensitisation threshold from "stressed but coping" to "systems offline." The infection was the trigger, but the chronic stress was what had depleted his buffer capacity. When the next crisis hit, there was nothing left to absorb it.

This is what I mean when I say fatigue is a production problem. James did not lack motivation. He didn't lack discipline. His mitochondria lacked fuel. His methylation was impaired. His gut was producing neurotoxins. His glutathione was depleted. And his testosterone had collapsed as a downstream consequence of all four. Every practitioner who told him to rest more and manage stress better was treating the symptom while the machinery continued to break down.

The Biochemistry Sequence

Just as gut restoration follows a five-phase sequence, biochemistry restoration has its own order. Just as in the gut chapter, the order matters as much as the interventions. Supporting mitochondria while Clostridia is producing neurotoxins is like pouring fuel into an engine that is being actively sabotaged. Restoring methylation while glutathione is depleted means the methylation products have nowhere safe to go. Adding testosterone support while the upstream biochemistry is broken means the testosterone will not hold, because the systems that maintain it are still offline.

The first step is clearing gut interference. If the organic acids test shows elevated Clostridia markers, yeast metabolites, or bacterial overgrowth markers, these must be addressed before the biochemistry can stabilise. Herbal antimicrobials and targeted probiotics are the primary tools. This step often overlaps with or follows the gut repair protocol from the previous chapter. In James's case, the Clostridia clearance was the highest priority, because as long as those bacteria were producing neurotoxins, no amount of dopamine support or methylation supplementation would hold.

The second step is restoring methylation. Once gut interference is being addressed, methylation support can begin. A methylated B-complex provides the active forms of folate and B12 that bypass common genetic bottlenecks such as MTHFR variants. SAMe (S-adenosylmethionine) is the body's primary methyl donor, and in cases of significant undermethylation, targeted SAMe supplementation can accelerate the restoration. The goal is to bring homocysteine down into the optimal range, which signals that the methylation cycle is turning over efficiently. For James, this meant moving homocysteine from 14.8 to below 7.

The third step is rebuilding glutathione. NAC (N-acetyl cysteine) provides the rate-limiting amino acid for glutathione production. Glycine, the second amino acid in the glutathione molecule, is often co-supplemented. Alpha-lipoic acid recycles glutathione and supports mitochondrial function directly. This step restores the body's antioxidant defence, protects the mitochondria from oxidative damage, and reopens the detoxification pathways that have been backed up.

The fourth step is supporting mitochondrial function directly. CoQ10 is the critical cofactor for the electron transport chain. The final stage of ATP production. Magnesium supports ATP synthesis and over three hundred enzymatic reactions. B vitamins fuel the Krebs cycle at multiple steps. PQQ (pyrroloquinoline quinone) supports the growth of new mitochondria. And acetyl-L-carnitine transports fatty acids into the mitochondria for fuel. These interventions are only fully effective once the upstream problems, gut interference, methylation, and glutathione, have been addressed. Adding CoQ10 to a patient with active Clostridia and depleted glutathione is like adding premium fuel to an engine that is overheating and leaking oil.

The fifth step, and the one that most practitioners reach for first, is hormonal support. For James, this meant zinc, adaptogens, and testosterone supporting herbs to aid recovery. But this step came last, not first. Because testosterone is downstream. It is produced and maintained by systems that depend on adequate methylation, functioning detoxification, healthy gut ecology, and sufficient mitochondrial energy. Treat those upstream systems, and the testosterone often recovers without direct hormonal intervention. In James's case, that is exactly what happened.

What Happened with James

James's protocol followed the sequence. We cleared the Clostridia with targeted antimicrobials and soil-based probiotics over the first twelve weeks. In parallel, we began methylation support with a methylated B-complex and SAMe, and started rebuilding glutathione with NAC and glycine. Once the gut interference was clearing and the detoxification pathways were reopening, we introduced mitochondrial support: CoQ10, magnesium, B vitamins, and acetyl-L-carnitine. Testosterone support, zinc, and adaptogenic herbs were introduced last, after the upstream systems were stable.

At eight months, we retested.

Glutathione markers had normalised. Aconitic acid and pyroglutamic acid were both within the healthy range. His cellular defence system was back online. Clostridia markers had cleared, the neurotoxin production had stopped. HVA, his dopamine precursor marker, had returned to the healthy range. Homocysteine had dropped from 14.8 to 6.2 — optimal. His methylation pathway was functioning. And testosterone had risen from 265 to 550 ng/dL, more than doubling without testosterone replacement therapy. The upstream repair had allowed the downstream system to recover on its own.

James described feeling clear, capable, and resilient again. Not wired. Not driven by adrenaline or caffeine. His energy was steady through the day. His brain fog had lifted. His concentration had returned. His mood had stabilised naturally as the neurotransmitter pathways came back online. His exercise tolerance improved and he was training again without the post-exercise crashes that had plagued him for three years. He no longer looked like someone who was coping. For the first time in years, he did not need to.

He did not need to slow down. He needed his biochemistry restored. The burnout was real, but it was not the cause. It was the consequence of a biochemical cascade that started with chronic stress, was triggered by an infection, and expressed itself as energy failure, hormonal collapse, and cognitive decline. Once the cascade was reversed in sequence, the systems came back online in the order they were designed to operate.

This is the second layer of the restoration sequence. The gut comes first because it controls absorption, immune function, and the microbial environment that either supports or sabotages everything downstream. Biochemistry comes second because it translates nutrients into function — energy, detoxification, neurotransmitter production, hormonal support. If the gut is the gatekeeper, biochemistry is the engine. Fix the gatekeeper, and the engine can receive fuel. Fix the engine, and the body can produce the output it needs to function, recover, and perform.

James's case hinged on recognising that his fatigue was not one problem but a cascade — mitochondrial, methylation, gut-driven, and hormonal, each feeding the others. The framework identified the sequence. But the clinical precision was knowing which cofactors to start, which to delay until detox capacity improved, and when to shift from biochemical restoration to hormonal support. This came from interpreting the pattern across all three tests at once. That integration is where generic supplement protocols diverge from sequenced recovery.

Hormones come third, and the next chapter explains why — a different patient, a different pattern. The same principle: downstream systems cannot stabilise until the upstream drivers are addressed. Sequence determines outcome.

JAMES — Burnout & Testosterone Recovery (8 months)

MARKER	BEFORE		AFTER
Total Testosterone	265 ng/dL	→	550 ng/dL
Homocysteine	14.8 µmol/L	→	6.2 µmol/L
Pyroglutamic Acid	Elevated	→	Normal
Vitamin B6	Low	→	Optimised
Clostridia Markers	Elevated	→	Cleared
HVA (Dopamine)	Low	→	Normal

Energy restored. Testosterone doubled without TRT. Brain fog lifted.

James's protocol breakdown is available at TheHealingHierarchy.com.

His body hadn't been failing. Its machinery had been blocked.

Chapter Twelve

Hormones Are Downstream

Emma had done everything right. She ate well. She exercised. She tracked her calories. She followed the advice she had been given after her first child was born: get back on track, lose the baby weight, push through the fatigue. And for a while, she managed. But by her mid-thirties, her body had stopped cooperating.

The fatigue was not the tired-after-a-bad-night kind. It was a bone-deep exhaustion that no amount of sleep could touch. She was gaining weight despite eating less than she ever had. She was cold all the time — hands, feet, core. Her hair was falling out in clumps. Her periods, once regular, had become unpredictable — lighter, shorter, further apart. Her mood had flattened into a persistent low-grade anxiety she had never experienced before. And when she brought up the anxiety, she was handed an SSRI prescription.

She had been diagnosed with Hashimoto's thyroiditis. An autoimmune condition in which the immune system attacks the thyroid gland. She was told it was manageable with medication and monitoring. She was put on thyroid hormone replacement. It helped slightly. Her TSH improved on paper. But the fatigue remained. The weight stayed. The hair loss continued. The periods did not normalise. And the harder she pushed, cutting more calories, increasing exercise intensity, the worse everything got. Her body had entered what I call siege mode: perceiving restriction and stress as survival threats, it slowed metabolism, raised cortisol, held onto weight, and refused to release it no matter how compliant she was.

At some point, she had stopped expecting things to improve. She still went through the motions, the appointments, the supplements, the early-morning walks, but without the belief that any of it would change the trajectory. She had accepted that this was simply what her body did now.

When she came to my clinic, she expected me to adjust her thyroid medication. Instead, I told her that her thyroid was not the problem. It was the messenger.

The Thyroid Is a Network

The previous two chapters established the first two layers of the restoration sequence: the gut as the gatekeeper, biochemistry as the engine. Hormones are the third layer, and the most common place where both patients and practitioners start. It is also, in most cases, the wrong place to start. Hormones are downstream. They are the output of systems that sit above them in the hierarchy. When those upstream systems - gut integrity, nutrient status, methylation, detoxification, inflammation - are compromised, the hormonal system can't function properly. Treating hormones without fixing the upstream drivers is like adjusting the heating or cooling in a house with broken windows. The setting changes. The temperature does not.

The thyroid is the clearest example of this principle. Most patients who present with thyroid symptoms have been tested with a single marker: TSH, thyroid stimulating hormone. TSH is a pituitary hormone, not a thyroid hormone. A signal sent from the brain to the thyroid gland telling it how much hormone to produce. It is useful as a screening tool. It is entirely inadequate as a diagnostic one. A normal TSH does not mean the thyroid is functioning well. It means the pituitary is satisfied with the signal it is receiving. But it tells you nothing about whether the thyroid gland is producing adequate amounts of T4, whether T4 is being converted into the active form T3, whether reverse T3 is blocking the receptors, or whether the immune system is attacking the gland itself.

A full thyroid assessment requires TSH, free T4, free T3, reverse T3, TPO antibodies, and thyroglobulin antibodies. Without all six, you are looking at the thyroid through a keyhole. Optimal TSH is between 0.4 and 2.0 mIU/L. Not the laboratory range that extends to 4.5 or even 5.0. Free T4 should sit between 14 and 20 pmol/L. Free T3, the active hormone that drives cellular metabolism, should be between 4.0 and 5.5 pmol/L. TPO antibodies above 34 IU/mL and thyroglobulin antibodies above 115 IU/mL indicate autoimmune thyroid disease. I have picked up dozens of cases where TSH was technically within the laboratory range but the full panel revealed Hashimoto's, poor T4-to-T3 conversion, or elevated reverse T3 blocking the active hormone from reaching the cells.

But the thyroid panel alone is still not enough. The thyroid doesn't operate in isolation. It requires selenium for T4-to-T3 conversion. It requires zinc for thyroid receptor sensitivity. It requires iodine as a raw material for thyroid hormone production. It requires adequate iron for thyroid peroxidase enzyme activity. It requires stable cortisol, because chronic stress suppresses thyroid output directly through the HPA axis.

Beyond those cofactors, the thyroid depends on systems that most practitioners never assess alongside a thyroid panel. It requires a healthy gut, because intestinal permeability drives the autoimmune process through molecular mimicry, where the immune system confuses food proteins, particularly gluten, with thyroid tissue.

Alessio Fasano's research on zonulin, the protein that regulates tight junction permeability, established that intestinal permeability is not merely a symptom of autoimmune disease but a prerequisite for its development. His triad model identifies three conditions required for autoimmunity: genetic susceptibility, an environmental trigger, and increased intestinal permeability. Emma had all three. It requires functioning detoxification pathways, because if the body can't clear excess oestrogen, oestrogen dominance blocks thyroid receptors and worsens every thyroid symptom.

This is why thyroid medication alone so often fails to resolve the full symptom picture. The medication replaces the hormone. It does nothing to address why the gland was underperforming, why the immune system is attacking it, why the conversion pathways are impaired, or why the cofactors are depleted. The prescription replaces what the body isn't producing without asking why it stopped.

Autoimmunity Is a Signal, Not a Sentence

Hashimoto's thyroiditis is the most common autoimmune condition in the developed world, and it accounts for the majority of hypothyroid cases I see in clinic. The conventional framing is that the immune system has malfunctioned. That it is mistakenly attacking the thyroid gland, and that this attack must be managed with hormone replacement and monitoring. That framing is incomplete.

In my clinical experience, the immune system in Hashimoto's is not malfunctioning. It is responding to a trigger it cannot resolve. The same principle that applied to Sarah's autoimmunity in Chapter 10 applies here: the immune activation is the symptom, not the cause. Something upstream is driving the attack. In the majority of Hashimoto's cases I see, that something is gut permeability combined with one or more of the following: chronic inflammation, nutrient depletion, food-driven immune reactivity, or hormonal imbalance.

The mechanism is well-established. When the intestinal barrier is compromised — leaky gut — partially digested food proteins, bacterial fragments, and toxins cross into the bloodstream. The immune system mounts a response. In genetically susceptible individuals, the immune system then begins to cross-react: it identifies structural similarities between the foreign proteins and the body's own tissues. Gluten is the most well-documented trigger for thyroid molecular mimicry. The gliadin protein in gluten shares structural features with thyroid tissue, and the immune system, already primed by gut-driven inflammation, begins targeting both. This isn't a permanent state. When the gut is repaired and the inflammatory triggers are removed, the immune activation can slow, and in many cases, the antibodies drop significantly.

Thyroid antibodies are a measure of immune activation against the thyroid. When the drivers are addressed — gut permeability sealed, inflammatory foods removed, mineral cofactors restored, detoxification pathways reopened — those antibodies can fall. I have seen drops of sixty, seventy, eighty per cent in patients who have been told their condition is permanent and progressive. It is only progressive if the upstream drivers are never addressed. It isn't inevitable.

The Hormone Cascade

Emma's case illustrates something critical that extends beyond the thyroid: hormones don't operate in isolation. They operate in a cascade, where each hormone influences and is influenced by the others. Understanding this cascade is essential for understanding why treating a single hormone in isolation rarely works.

The thyroid and sex hormones are directly connected. Low progesterone worsens thyroid function. High oestrogen blocks thyroid receptors, effectively preventing thyroid hormone from reaching the cells even when blood levels appear adequate. Oestrogen dominance, which can result from impaired detoxification, high beta-glucuronidase in the gut, chronic stress, or post-partum hormonal shifts, is one of the most common and most overlooked contributors to thyroid symptom persistence.

The thyroid and cortisol are directly connected. Chronic stress elevates cortisol, which suppresses TSH and impairs T4-to-T3 conversion. The body prioritises survival over metabolism. In a prolonged stress state, the body will downregulate thyroid output to conserve energy. A protective mechanism that becomes pathological when the stress does not resolve. This is why patients under chronic stress often present with subclinical hypothyroidism that doesn't fully respond to thyroid medication: the HPA axis is suppressing thyroid function as a survival strategy, and prescribed hormone alone cannot override that signal while the stress persists.

The thyroid and the gut are directly connected. The gut produces precursors for thyroid hormone synthesis. Low stomach acid, common in Hashimoto's, impairs absorption of iron, zinc, selenium, and B12, all of which are required for thyroid function. Gut dysbiosis and elevated beta-glucuronidase reactivate oestrogen that should have been cleared, feeding oestrogen dominance. Intestinal permeability drives the autoimmune process itself through molecular mimicry. This was precisely Emma's picture: beta-glucuronidase elevated, oestrogen recycling back into her system, thyroid receptors functionally blocked, and a gut barrier wide open sustaining the autoimmune fire. It is a self-perpetuating loop. A compromised gut drives the autoimmune attack on the thyroid, the thyroid dysfunction impairs gut motility and stomach acid production, and the resulting malabsorption worsens the nutrient deficiencies that the thyroid depends on. Without breaking this loop at the gut level, thyroid treatment remains a holding pattern.

Emma's Data

Emma's testing confirmed that her thyroid was responding to systemic pressure from every direction.

Her thyroid panel showed the autoimmune picture clearly. TPO antibodies were 485 IU/mL, normal is below 34. Thyroglobulin antibodies were 320 IU/mL, normal is below 115. Her immune system was launching a sustained assault on her thyroid gland. TSH was 4.8 mIU/L — technically within the laboratory reference range, but well above the optimal threshold of 2.0. Her free T3 and free T4 were both low-normal: the thyroid was producing some hormone, but not enough for adequate cellular energy, and what it was producing was not converting efficiently to the active form.

Her mineral status explained why. Selenium was low. The mineral most critical for T4-to-T3 conversion and for reducing thyroid antibodies. Zinc was low, required for thyroid receptor sensitivity. Iodine was low, but could not be supplemented yet, because iodine in the presence of active autoimmune thyroid disease and without adequate selenium is like pouring fuel on a fire. It accelerates the antibody attack rather than supporting the gland. And copper on hair tissue mineral analysis was elevated at 68 ppm against a normal range of 10 to 27, antagonising zinc and fuelling oxidative stress.

Her gut told the rest of the story. Zonulin was 196 — normal is below 107. Her intestinal barrier was wide open, allowing the immune triggers to cross into the bloodstream and sustain the autoimmune attack. Secretory IgA was low, her gut immune defence was compromised. And beta-glucuronidase was elevated, a marker showing that gut bacteria were reactivating oestrogen that should have been cleared through the liver and eliminated. That oestrogen was being recycled back into her system, feeding oestrogen dominance and blocking thyroid receptor function.

Her hormonal panel confirmed the downstream collapse. Day 21 progesterone was 12 nmol/L, optimal is above 30. Her luteal phase was failing. Progesterone was too low to balance oestrogen, support mood, or maintain a healthy menstrual cycle. Her periods had become irregular not because of a primary reproductive problem, but because the entire hormonal axis was being destabilised from upstream: autoimmune thyroid driving inflammation, gut permeability driving the autoimmune process, nutrient depletion starving the thyroid of cofactors, and impaired detoxification trapping oestrogen in her system.

Her OAT added the biochemical layer. Vitamin B6 was low. A critical cofactor for both progesterone production and liver detoxification. Pyroglutamic acid was elevated, meaning glutathione was depleted, confirming that her detoxification pathways were overwhelmed.

Post-partum thyroid flare combined with aggressive calorie restriction. Her body had entered siege mode — perceiving starvation and stress as survival threats. Her metabolism slowed, her thyroid antibodies surged, and her progesterone collapsed. And her body refused to release weight despite perfect compliance. This was not a failure of willpower. It was her body's survival response to perceived scarcity. The harder she pushed, the tighter her body held on.

The Intervention Sequence

Treating Emma's thyroid directly at this stage would have missed the point. Increasing her thyroid medication wouldn't address the autoimmune attack, the leaky gut feeding the immune fire, the mineral deficiencies blocking hormone conversion, the progesterone collapse, or the detox dysfunction trapping oestrogen. The priority was upstream. The intervention followed four phases — each building on the one before it.

Phase 1: Calm the fire. The first priority was reducing the immune and inflammatory burden driving the autoimmune attack using a gut repair formula containing L-glutamine and zinc carnosine, along with targeted probiotics to begin sealing the intestinal permeability that was sustaining the autoimmune process. An autoimmune protocol diet removed the primary immune triggers: gluten, dairy, grains, legumes, nightshades, eggs, nuts, seeds, refined sugars, and processed foods. In their place: organ meats, bone broth, wild-caught fish, pastured proteins, diverse non-nightshade vegetables, fermented foods, and healing fats. Selenium and zinc supplementation began immediately, selenium to support T4-to-T3 conversion and reduce antibodies, zinc to restore receptor sensitivity and oppose the elevated copper, along with molybdenum to support the detoxification pathways her body needed to clear the excess oestrogen and copper load.

Phase 2: Restore clearance. With the inflammatory load reduced, attention turned to the detoxification and clearance pathways that were trapping oestrogen in her system. Vitamin B6 in its active form, P-5-P, to support both progesterone synthesis and liver detoxification. Calcium-D-glucarate to block the elevated beta-glucuronidase and stop the oestrogen recycling. Methylation support followed: liposomal glutathione, NAC, and methylated B vitamins, to restore glutathione levels and reopen the detoxification pathways.

Phase 3: Rebuild hormonal production. With the gut stabilising and clearance pathways reopening, the body was now in a position to respond to hormonal support. Vitex, chaste tree berry, to stimulate pituitary signalling and support progesterone production in the luteal phase. Magnesium glycinate to calm the nervous system and support progesterone synthesis. Omega-3 fatty acids to reduce inflammation and support hormonal balance. Plus a critical lifestyle shift: reduced exercise intensity, from high-intensity training to walking and restorative movement, and improved sleep hygiene. Cortisol steals progesterone's precursors. Her chronic stress was actively suppressing the hormone her cycle most needed. Until the stress signal changed, her body couldn't rebuild what it had lost.

Phase 4: Cautious iodine trial. Iodine was deliberately avoided for the first six months. This is the decision that most practitioners get wrong with Hashimoto's. Iodine is essential for thyroid hormone production. The gland can't make it without this mineral. But in the presence of active autoimmune thyroid disease, iodine stimulates the very enzyme the antibodies are attacking. The relationship follows a U-shaped curve: too much worsens autoimmunity, but chronic deficiency also increases it. Both extremes cause harm. The answer sits in the middle — the right dose, at the right time, in the right patient.

Reintroduction is appropriate only when selenium has been supplemented for at least three months and confirmed adequate, TPO antibodies have dropped significantly, and gut permeability has been addressed. The dose must be low, 150 to 250 micrograms, and monitored with retesting at four to six weeks. If antibodies rise, iodine is withdrawn immediately. Some patients respond well. Others do not tolerate it regardless of how stable their upstream systems appear. The margin between therapeutic and harmful is narrow, and this isn't something patients should self-prescribe.

For Emma, the timing was right. After six months of upstream work, gut repair, mineral restoration, detoxification support, and immune calming, her antibodies had dropped sufficiently and her selenium had been restored. Low-dose iodine accelerated her recovery rather than sabotaging it. Had we started with iodine on day one, the outcome would have been very different.

What Happened with Emma

By month three, Emma's period had normalized: cycles returned to twenty-eight days and flow returned to healthy volume. PMS symptoms including mood swings, breast tenderness and the anxiety that had prompted the SSRI prescription, had dramatically reduced. Day 21 progesterone retested at 34 nmol/L. Optimal. Her luteal phase was functioning again.

Between months three and six, the systemic changes accumulated. Her energy became consistent, no more two o'clock crashes. Cold intolerance resolved, her hands and feet were warm again, and hair shedding reduced significantly with new growth becoming visible. Her anxiety softened. Her stress tolerance improved. And her weight stabilised without calorie restriction. Her body had finally come out of siege mode because it no longer perceived scarcity as the primary threat.

At nine months, we retested.

Thyroid antibodies had dropped by eighty per cent. TPO from 485 to 95. Thyroglobulin antibodies from 320 to 68 — within normal range. Emma's result sits at the higher end of what I see in practice, reductions of forty to sixty per cent are more typical within this timeframe, depending on the severity of the upstream drivers and how long the autoimmune process has been active. But the direction is consistent. When the drivers are addressed in sequence, antibodies fall. TSH had come down to 1.5. Free T3 and free T4 were in optimal range. Selenium, zinc, and iodine were all restored. Zonulin had dropped from 215 to 72 — her gut barrier was intact. Secretory IgA had restored. Beta-glucuronidase, B6, and glutathione markers had all normalised. The upstream systems were functioning. The downstream hormones had followed.

Emma had been told that Hashimoto's was a life sentence — something to manage, never resolve. She had been given medication for the output and told nothing about the input. Nobody had tested her gut. Nobody had measured her progesterone or her detoxification markers. Nobody had connected the autoimmune thyroid attack to the intestinal permeability, the oestrogen dominance, and the nutrient depletion that were driving it.

But the numbers were only part of the story. Somewhere between months three and nine, Emma had started expecting things to get better again. That shift, from giving up to taking control, was as important as anything the blood work showed.

We did not cure her Hashimoto's. The genetic susceptibility remains. But we removed the upstream drivers that were fuelling the autoimmune fire. When those drivers were addressed in sequence, the antibodies dropped, the thyroid recovered, the hormones rebalanced, and the symptoms that had defined her life for years resolved. Her body was not broken. It was overloaded. And when the load was reduced in the right order, it began to heal.

When Direct Hormonal Support Is Warranted

The principle of this chapter, fix upstream before treating downstream, is the foundation of how I approach every hormonal case. But it isn't an absolute. There are situations where upstream systems have been addressed, foundational work has been completed, natural support has been trialled, and the hormonal system still needs direct intervention. In those cases, hormonal support is the next appropriate step in the sequence.

The clinical principle is clear: replacement is appropriate when the gland can't recover, not when the system hasn't been assessed.

For women in later perimenopause and menopause, this is particularly relevant. I think of a patient I see regularly. A woman in her early fifties who had done the foundational work thoroughly: gut repaired, minerals balanced, detoxification functioning, stress managed. Her upstream systems were sound, but the ovarian decline was advanced enough that her body could no longer produce the oestrogen and progesterone it needed for sleep, cognitive clarity, and bone density. That is the profile where bioidentical hormones become not just reasonable but necessary.

The decline in oestrogen and progesterone during this transition is a natural biological shift. But when that shift produces symptoms that significantly impair quality of life — severe hot flushes, sleep disruption, bone density loss, cognitive changes, vaginal atrophy, mood instability, and when foundational work and herbal support have not been sufficient, bioidentical hormone replacement becomes a legitimate and often valuable option.

The distinction matters. Bioidentical hormones are structurally identical to the hormones the body produces naturally. They are derived from plant sources and compounded to match human oestradiol and progesterone at a molecular level. This is structurally different from synthetic hormones, such as conjugated equine oestrogens and synthetic progestins, which have a different molecular structure and a different risk profile. Much of the fear around hormone replacement stems from research conducted on synthetic formulations. The evidence on bioidentical hormones, when prescribed appropriately and monitored regularly, paints a different picture.

My clinical approach is sequential. First, address the upstream drivers — gut, inflammation, nutrient status, stress, detoxification. Second, trial natural hormonal support: Vitex for progesterone, phytoestrogenic herbs, adaptogenic herbs for adrenal and cortisol support, and lifestyle modifications including sleep optimisation and stress regulation. For many women, particularly in early perimenopause, this is sufficient. The body still has the capacity to produce adequate hormones when the systems supporting that production are functioning. But when natural approaches have been given adequate time and the symptoms persist, or when the hormonal decline is advanced enough that the body can no longer produce sufficient levels regardless of upstream support, bioidentical oestrogen and progesterone become the appropriate intervention. The principle is start low, go slow, and test regularly. Dosing is guided by symptoms and confirmed by blood or saliva hormone panels at regular intervals. The goal is the minimum effective dose that resolves symptoms while maintaining safe hormone levels.

For men, the conversation around testosterone replacement requires a different framework. James's case in the previous chapter demonstrated that testosterone can recover significantly, from 265 to 550 ng/dL, without replacement therapy, simply by addressing the upstream drivers: clearing gut interference, restoring methylation, rebuilding glutathione, and supporting mitochondrial function. In my clinical opinion, testosterone replacement therapy should be a last resort for men, not a first-line intervention, with one exception: when there is confirmed testicular damage or primary output failure, TRT may be appropriate earlier in the sequence because the gland itself can't produce adequate hormone regardless of upstream support. Too often I see men placed on TRT before anyone has assessed their gut, their methylation status, their Clostridia load, their nutrient cofactors, or their sleep. Once TRT is started, the body's own production often shuts down, making it difficult to discontinue. That is a significant commitment, and it should only be made after the upstream systems have been thoroughly addressed and natural support has been given an adequate trial.

Natural testosterone support includes zinc, magnesium, and adequate sleep as foundational requirements. Vitamin D is also critical for testosterone production, but I prefer patients to obtain it from regular sun exposure first — fifteen to twenty minutes of direct sunlight on exposed skin most days is the most effective and bioavailable source. Supplementation is warranted when sun exposure is genuinely insufficient due to climate, lifestyle, or confirmed low levels on blood testing, but it isn't my first recommendation. Beyond those, herbal support such as tongkat ali, fadogia agrestis, and tribulus terrestris can provide meaningful additional support for men whose upstream systems have been stabilised but whose testosterone remains suboptimal. These are trialled after the foundational biochemistry work, not instead of it. If natural support and upstream restoration together do not produce adequate testosterone recovery, confirmed by retesting, then TRT becomes a reasonable and clinically justified option. But it is the end of the sequence, not the beginning. The same principle that governs this entire book applies: exhaust the upstream solutions before committing to downstream replacement.

This is what it means to say that hormones are downstream. The thyroid did not fail on its own. It was undermined by a leaky gut, starved of cofactors, attacked by an immune system responding to triggers it couldn't clear, and destabilised by a hormonal cascade in which every system was pulling the others down. Treating the thyroid without fixing the gut, restoring the minerals, calming the immune activation, and rebalancing the hormonal axis would have been a permanent holding pattern, managing the symptoms while the systems driving them continued to deteriorate.

The gut is the gatekeeper. Biochemistry is the engine. Hormones are the output. Fix them in that order, and the body does what it was designed to do.

When you treat hormones first, you manage decline. When you restore the systems above them, you allow recovery.

Emma's recovery required restraint as much as intervention. The decision to delay iodine for six months, to prioritise gut repair before hormonal support, and to address the oestrogen recycling pathway before touching the thyroid medication. Those decisions are counterintuitive. They require understanding not just what each marker means, but how each intervention will interact with a system that is already sensitised. For uncomplicated hormonal cases, the framework in this chapter gives you the roadmap. For complex autoimmune-thyroid presentations like Emma's, the roadmap benefits from a guide who has walked it before.

The next chapter turns to the fourth system in the sequence: mood, anxiety, and neurotransmitters. A different patient. A different pattern. The same architecture, and the same discovery that what looks like a psychological problem is often a biological one with a biochemical cause.

EMMA — Hashimoto's & Hormonal Restoration (9 months)

MARKER	BEFORE		AFTER
TPO Antibodies	485 IU/mL	→	~95 IU/mL
Thyroglobulin Ab	320 IU/mL	→	Reduced
Free T3	Low	→	Optimised
Progesterone (Day 21)	12 nmol/L	→	Normalised
Beta-glucuronidase	Elevated	→	Normalised
Zonulin	Elevated	→	Restored

Antibodies dropped 80%. Hormonal cycles stabilised. Medication reduced.

Emma's protocol breakdown is available at TheHealingHierarchy.com.

The thyroid was never the problem. It was the first place the damage became really visible.

Chapter Thirteen

What Looks Like a Mind Problem Is Usually a Brain Problem

Alex's mum sat across from me, exhausted and worried.

"Everyone keeps telling us it's just university stress," she said. "But I know my son. This isn't normal."

Alex was twenty-one, in his third year of university. On paper, he should have been thriving. He was at a good school, had a supportive family, and no major trauma. But over the past eighteen months, something had shifted. The anxiety had become constant, not situational nerves before an exam, but a background hum of dread that never went away. He was having panic attacks: heart racing, chest tight, the feeling that he was dying. His thoughts raced. He could read the same paragraph five times and retain nothing. Sleep had collapsed, it took two to three hours to fall asleep, waking multiple times, energy drinks to get through the day. He had quietly stopped hanging out with friends, quit the soccer team (a sport he had played since high school), and watched his grades slide from B-plus to barely passing.

He had tried university counselling. It helped with stress management techniques but did not touch the physical symptoms. His GP ran a standard blood panel, full blood count, iron studies, basic thyroid, and everything came back within normal limits. The GP prescribed an SSRI. It made him feel numb and disconnected — he stopped after three weeks. He tried meditation apps but could not sit still long enough for them to work. He drank more coffee, which made the anxiety worse. He was caught in a cycle where every intervention either failed or amplified the problem.

His mum was worried he would drop out. Alex was worried he was broken.

"He's always been a sensitive kid," she said. "But this is different. He's not himself."

She was right. He wasn't himself. But the reason had nothing to do with his psychology. It had everything to do with his biochemistry.

The Brain Is an Organ

The previous three chapters established the restoration sequence: gut as gatekeeper, biochemistry as engine, hormones as output. This chapter addresses the fourth system, and the one most commonly misdiagnosed: mood, anxiety, and neurotransmitter function. The conventional model often treats these primarily as psychological problems. In my clinical experience, they are usually biological problems with a biochemical cause.

The brain is an organ. It has metabolic requirements just like every other organ in the body. It requires nutrients to produce neurotransmitters, a functioning gut to supply precursors, and stable blood sugar to maintain energy. It requires adequate methylation to synthesise the chemicals that regulate mood, focus, sleep, and emotional stability. When any of these upstream systems are compromised, the brain's neurochemistry changes, and the result looks exactly like a mental health disorder. The symptoms are real. They aren't imagined. But they are the end result, not the cause. If you treat the result without investigating what is driving it, you get what Alex got: medication that numbs the signal without addressing what is generating it.

Your Brain Cannot Make Calm Without Raw Materials

The brain produces two broad categories of neurotransmitters: inhibitory and excitatory. The inhibitory neurotransmitters, serotonin and GABA, calm the nervous system. Serotonin promotes stable mood, well-being, connection, and healthy sleep-wake cycles. It also regulates bowel motility, pain perception, and carbohydrate cravings. GABA balances excitation, enhances focus, and allows the mind to switch off at night. When serotonin is low, the result is depression, constipation, waking through the night, poor pain management, and cravings. When GABA is low, the result is anxiety, racing thoughts, the inability to calm down, and insomnia.

The excitatory neurotransmitters, dopamine, noradrenaline, and adrenaline, drive motivation, alertness, focus, and the stress response. Dopamine is the reward and motivation chemical; low levels are linked to addiction, ADHD, and the flat, joyless state that gets labelled depression when it is actually a dopamine production deficit. Noradrenaline drives attention and action. Adrenaline powers the fight-or-flight response. These neurotransmitters need to be in balance, not too much, not too little.

Here is what most practitioners miss: the brain can't produce these neurotransmitters without specific nutrient cofactors. Tryptophan converts to serotonin, but only in the presence of B6, zinc, and folate. Tyrosine converts to dopamine, but only when methylation is functioning and iron is adequate. The biopterin pathway, which is the master switch for both serotonin and dopamine production, requires folate, iron, and tetrahydrobiopterin. If any of these cofactors are depleted, the conversion pathways stall. The brain has the raw amino acid precursors but cannot assemble them into functioning neurotransmitters.

Here is the fundamental error in the SSRI model. SSRIs work by blocking the reuptake of serotonin — keeping more serotonin active in the synapse. But if the brain isn't producing adequate serotonin in the first place, there is nothing to keep in the synapse. The medication is designed to recycle a chemical that the brain can't manufacture.

It is like installing a more efficient drainage system in a house where the taps are not running.

The Gut-Brain Axis

Chapter 10 established that the gut is the gatekeeper. What that chapter did not fully explore is the gut's direct role in brain function. Ninety per cent of the body's serotonin is produced in the gastrointestinal tract, not in the brain. Gut bacteria produce precursors for serotonin, GABA, and dopamine. The gut and brain communicate directly through the vagus nerve. A bidirectional highway where information flows in both directions. When the gut microbiome is disrupted, the brain's neurochemistry changes.

This is measurable and testable. Gut dysbiosis, particularly overgrowth of Clostridia species, produces neurotoxins such as HPHPA and 4-cresol that directly interfere with dopamine and GABA signalling. James's case in Chapter 11 showed how Clostridia markers on his OAT explained fatigue and low motivation. The same mechanism drives anxiety, brain fog, and mood instability. A compromised gut doesn't just cause digestive problems. It alters brain chemistry directly.

The gut-brain connection runs deeper still. Intestinal permeability, the leaky gut that Sarah's case demonstrated in Chapter 10, allows bacterial endotoxins into the bloodstream. These endotoxins cross the blood-brain barrier and trigger neuroinflammation. Chronic low-grade brain inflammation produces symptoms that are clinically indistinguishable from depression: flat mood, fatigue, withdrawal, cognitive slowing, loss of interest. The patient presents as depressed. The GP prescribes an antidepressant. But the driver is inflammatory, not psychological, and no antidepressant can resolve an inflammatory process originating in the gut.

Two Hidden Drivers

Beyond neurotransmitter synthesis and the gut-brain axis, two additional upstream drivers commonly present as mood disorders: blood sugar instability and chronic inflammation.

Blood sugar volatility is one of the most underdiagnosed contributors to anxiety and panic. Reactive hypoglycaemia - where blood sugar spikes after a high-carbohydrate meal and then crashes below baseline — triggers an adrenaline surge as the body attempts to stabilise glucose levels. The patient experiences heart palpitations, sweating, trembling, a sense of impending doom. It feels exactly like a panic attack. Because it is a panic attack, but the trigger is metabolic, not psychological. Alex's daily energy drink habit was doing exactly this — spiking glucose, then triggering an adrenaline surge that he and his GP were calling anxiety. The patient is told they have an anxiety disorder. What they have is a blood sugar regulation problem that can be addressed through dietary modification: protein-rich meals, reduced refined carbohydrates, and stable eating patterns that prevent the spike-crash cycle.

Chronic inflammation is the other hidden driver. Inflammation is metabolically expensive. It diverts resources away from neurotransmitter production, consumes B vitamins and zinc, depletes glutathione, and directly impairs brain function through the neuroinflammatory pathways described above. Alex's CRP would come back at 2.8 mg/L, more than double the optimal threshold, confirming an inflammatory burden that his brain couldn't ignore. The inflammation does not cause sadness in the way a life event does. It creates a biological state: fatigue, withdrawal, cognitive dulling, and loss of interest that the patient and the clinician interpret as depression. Address the inflammation, through gut repair, dietary change, and targeted anti-inflammatory support, and the "depression" often lifts without a single psychiatric intervention.

Biochemical Patterns Behind Mental Health

The work of Dr William Walsh, author of *Nutrient Power*, has been foundational in my approach to mood and anxiety. Walsh's research, spanning decades and tens of thousands of patients, identified distinct biochemical patterns that underlie mental health disorders. These are not personality types. They are measurable, testable biochemical profiles that dictate which nutrients the brain needs and which interventions will work.

These patterns are not mutually exclusive. A single patient can carry two or three simultaneously, which is what Alex did, and why his neurochemical disruption was so severe.

Undermethylation is the most common pattern I see in clinic. Undermethylators cannot efficiently produce SAMe, the universal methyl donor that the brain requires for serotonin and dopamine synthesis. They tend to be perfectionistic, high-achieving, and internally tense. Histamine is typically elevated, which drives racing thoughts and hyperarousal. Serotonin and dopamine are low. Not because of reuptake problems, but because the brain cannot manufacture enough. This is why undermethylators often respond poorly to SSRIs: the problem is not serotonin recycling, it is serotonin production. The intervention is methylated B vitamins, SAMe, zinc, and B6 — the cofactors the methylation cycle needs to function.

Pyrrole disorder is the second pattern, and it frequently overlaps with undermethylation. Elevated kryptopyrroles, waste products from haemoglobin synthesis, bind to B6 and zinc and pull them out of the body through urine. This creates a chronic, relentless depletion that can't be corrected through diet alone. The clinical signs are distinctive: morning nausea, poor dream recall, white spots on fingernails, stretch marks despite stable weight, sensitivity to light, inner tension, and mood swings. The patient loses the two nutrients most critical for neurotransmitter production faster than the body can replace them. Without targeted high-dose B6 and zinc supplementation, the depletion is self-perpetuating.

Copper overload is the third pattern. Elevated copper relative to zinc drives anxiety, racing thoughts, and emotional reactivity. Copper amplifies excitatory neurotransmitter activity while suppressing dopamine and GABA. Zinc supplementation gradually restores the ratio, and the anxiety often resolves as the balance normalises.

Testing is specific: homocysteine, whole blood histamine, serum zinc, serum copper, kryptopyrroles, and vitamin B6 functional markers on the OAT. Once identified, each pattern has a targeted intervention. But they require testing, not guessing.

Alex's Data

Alex's testing revealed the collision of multiple biochemical patterns — each one sufficient to cause anxiety on its own, all of them operating at once.

His nutrient status was severely depleted. Functional B6 markers on the OAT were critically abnormal: xanthurenate at 85 µg/mg creatinine against a normal range below 40, with quinolinate also elevated. These markers confirmed that even if serum B6 appeared adequate, his body couldn't use it. A functional deficiency that standard blood testing would have missed entirely, and the reason his GP's blood panel had returned normal. Zinc was 8.9 µmol/L against an optimal range of 12 to 18, severely depleted. Copper was elevated at 29 µmol/L, driving excitatory dominance. Serum B12 was 185 pmol/L, below even the laboratory threshold of 200 and far below the optimal level of 500. Ferritin was 22 ng/mL, low iron stores, impairing oxygen delivery to the brain. Vitamin D was 32 nmol/L against an optimal range above 80, deficient.

His methylation and pyrrole markers confirmed the biochemical biotype. Homocysteine was 12.4 µmol/L, optimal is 5 to 7, confirming that his methylation pathways were sluggish. Whole blood histamine was elevated, consistent with the classic undermethylator pattern: internally driven anxiety, perfectionism, hyperarousal. Kryptopyrroles were elevated, confirming pyrrole disorder. The reason his B6 and zinc were chronically depleted despite reasonable dietary intake. His body was losing these nutrients through urine faster than he could replace them. Every clinical sign of pyrrole disorder was present: morning nausea, poor dream recall, white spots on his nails, stretch marks, light sensitivity, and the internal tension that his mother recognised as different from ordinary stress.

His gut confirmed the neurochemical disruption: Lactobacillus was low — the bacteria most associated with serotonin precursor production. Clostridia species were elevated, producing neurotoxins that directly interfere with dopamine and GABA signalling. Bifidobacterium was low — compromising the gut-brain axis and immune regulation.

His OAT completed the picture. HVA, the dopamine metabolite, was very low, confirming that his brain wasn't producing adequate dopamine. 5-HIAA, the serotonin metabolite, was low, confirming impaired serotonin synthesis. Pyroglutamic acid was 41.5 against a normal range below 28, glutathione was severely depleted, meaning his detoxification system was overwhelmed. And CRP, the chronic low-grade inflammation consuming nutrients and driving oxidative stress, was 2.8 mg/L against an optimal range below 1.0.

The Restoration Sequence

Alex's sensitisation threshold had been crossed gradually. He had always had the genetic vulnerability — the undermethylation, the pyrrole tendency. But the combination of university stress, chronic sleep deprivation, campus food devoid of zinc and B6, excessive caffeine, and no exercise had systematically depleted every buffer his body had. The anxiety that had always been manageable became unmanageable not because the stress increased beyond a critical point, but because his biochemical capacity to handle any stress at all had collapsed.

His recovery followed the same principle that has governed every case in this book: fix the upstream systems first, and the downstream symptoms resolve. The sequence was built in layers, each phase creating the conditions for the next.

Phase 1: Stabilise the foundation. Blood sugar regulation came first — protein-rich breakfast every morning, elimination of energy drinks, reduced refined carbohydrates, and stable eating patterns with no meal-skipping. Gut repair began in parallel: antimicrobials targeting the elevated Clostridia, followed by probiotics emphasising Lactobacillus and Bifidobacterium strains, and gut-healing foods where accessible — fermented foods, bone broth, zinc-rich snacks. Sleep hygiene was enforced: magnesium glycinate and L-theanine thirty minutes before bed, screens off by ten, and a minimum target of seven hours.

Phase 2: Restore the depleted cofactors. High-dose P-5-P, the active form of B6, to bypass the functional deficiency. Zinc picolinate to restore levels and oppose elevated copper. Iron bisglycinate for the depleted ferritin. Methylcobalamin for the functionally insufficient B12. Vitamin D to correct the deficiency. These are the raw materials the brain needs to build neurotransmitters. Without them, no amount of therapy, medication, or lifestyle modification can restore neurochemical function.

Phase 3: Restore methylation and neurotransmitter synthesis. SAMe as a direct methyl donor. The molecule Alex's undermethylation prevented him from producing efficiently. Folinic acid rather than folic acid. An alternative folate pathway better suited to undermethylators. Continued zinc, B6, and methylated B vitamins to sustain the cofactor supply as the methylation cycle restarted.

Phase 4: Rebuild glutathione and detoxification capacity. NAC twice daily as a glutathione precursor. Glycine to support both glutathione synthesis and provide a calming neurotransmitter effect. Alpha-lipoic acid for antioxidant support. Vitamin C to support the detoxification pathways. This phase addressed the pyroglutamic acid elevation. The depleted glutathione that was leaving his system unable to clear oxidative stress.

Phase 5: Neurotransmitter precursors — last, not first. Only after the gut was clearing, the cofactors were rebuilding, and the methylation cycle was restarting did we introduce direct neurotransmitter precursors. 5-HTP before bed to support serotonin production for sleep and mood. L-tyrosine in the morning to support dopamine production for focus and motivation. These were added at week eight, not week one. This sequencing is critical and it is the mistake most practitioners make with mood support.

Precursors Are Bridges, Not Crutches

The supplement industry sells 5-HTP and L-tyrosine as if they are standalone solutions for mood and focus. They aren't. They are precursors — raw materials that the brain must still process through enzymatic pathways that require B6, zinc, folate, iron, and functioning methylation. Giving a patient 5-HTP when their B6 is depleted is like delivering bricks to a construction site that has no builders. The raw material sits there. Nothing gets assembled.

This is why so many people try 5-HTP for mood or L-tyrosine for focus and report that "it didn't work." It didn't work because the cofactors required to convert those precursors into functioning neurotransmitters were missing. The precursor needs the enzymatic machinery. The enzymatic machinery needs the nutrients. The nutrients need a functioning gut to absorb them and adequate methylation to activate them. Cut the chain at any point and the precursor is useless.

In my clinical approach, neurotransmitter precursors are always a later intervention, never the first. They are bridges — temporary support that accelerates recovery while the underlying systems rebuild. Once the cofactors are rebalanced, the methylation cycle is functioning, and the gut is producing precursors naturally, most patients can taper the supplemental precursors without symptom return. The body takes over. That is recovery, not dependency.

What Happened with Alex

The first change came within six weeks. Alex's panic attacks stopped. Not reduced — stopped. The background hum of dread that had been constant for eighteen months began to lift. He described it as the volume being turned down on something he had not realised was always playing.

By week ten, his focus had returned. He could sit through lectures and retain information without rereading every paragraph. His racing thoughts had quieted. By month three, the morning nausea was gone, his sleep had normalised, and he described a clarity of thinking he had not experienced since high school. By month four, his anxiety was eighty-five per cent reduced. By month five, his grades had improved from barely passing to A's and B's. He had rejoined the soccer team. He was seeing his friends again.

His follow-up labs at five months confirmed the biochemical restoration. Homocysteine had dropped from 12.4 to 6.8 µmol/L, methylation restored and Xanthurenate had normalised at 28 µg/mg, indicating functional B6 deficiency was corrected. Zinc had risen from 8.9 to 13.8 µmol/L. Copper had normalised at 17 µmol/L, the copper-to-zinc ratio was much more balanced. B12 had reached 485 pmol/L. Ferritin was 82 ng/mL. Vitamin D was 118 nmol/L. Pyroglutamic acid had normalized indicating glutathione status was restored. HVA and 5-HIAA, the dopamine and serotonin metabolites, were both in healthy range. CRP had dropped from 2.8 to 0.7 mg/L. The inflammation had resolved.

His mum said: "We got our son back. We didn't realise how much he was suffering. We thought it was just university."

Alex said something that has stayed with me: "I thought my brain was just wired to be anxious. I didn't know I could feel this calm. I didn't know life could feel this easy."

He had not needed a different medication. He had not needed more therapy. He had needed his biochemistry restored so that his brain could manufacture the neurochemistry it was designed to produce. The anxiety was real, the panic attacks were real, the suffering was real. But the cause was not psychological. It was nutritional, biochemical, and gut-driven, and once those drivers were addressed in sequence, the symptoms that had been labelled an anxiety disorder resolved.

This is the pattern that connects every chapter in this section. Sarah's autoimmunity was driven by her gut. James's fatigue was driven by his biochemistry. Emma's thyroid was driven by everything upstream of it. And Alex's anxiety was driven by nutrient depletion, methylation failure, gut dysbiosis, and inflammation — all converging on a brain that couldn't produce the chemicals it needed to function.

When mood disorders are treated as character flaws, people suffer unnecessarily. When they are treated as biological patterns, they become solvable.

The approach does not change. The body does.

Test it. Sequence it. Restore it.

Alex's case is a clear example of how biochemical drivers can be identified and addressed in sequence. But his case also required clinical judgment that extended beyond the data: the decision to treat the Clostridia first despite the methylation findings, the choice to withhold direct serotonin support until the gut environment improved, and the management of the Herxheimer reaction at week two that nearly caused him to stop.

The next chapter turns to the final piece of the clinical picture: what happens when you have done the foundational work, addressed the upstream systems, and need to build a recovery plan that holds over time. That is where the protocol becomes a practice, and where short-term intervention becomes long-term resilience.

ALEX — Anxiety & Neurotransmitter Restoration (5 months)

MARKER	BEFORE		AFTER
Pyrroles	Elevated	→	Normalised
Zinc	Low	→	Optimised
Vitamin B6	Low	→	Optimised
Copper : Zinc Ratio	Imbalanced	→	Balanced
Clostridia (HPHPA)	Elevated	→	Cleared
HVA / VMA	Depleted	→	Restored

Panic attacks stopped. Sleep normalised. Came off SSRI under supervision.

Alex's protocol breakdown is available at TheHealingHierarchy.com.

The cause was biochemical. And the biochemical cause had a sequence.

PART V
PROTOCOLS AND ADJUSTMENT

Chapter Fourteen

Protocols Are Not Permanent

I will call her Kate. She came to see me eighteen months after her initial recovery. She had been a patient with excellent outcomes — gut repaired, energy restored, thyroid stable, mood balanced. Her data had been clean across every marker. She left my clinic feeling better than she had in a decade. And then she stopped everything.

She stopped the probiotics and the methylated B vitamins, reintroduced gluten and dairy without structure. She stopped tracking her sleep. She assumed that because she felt well, the job was done. Within six months, her symptoms were returning, not all at once, but in a pattern anyone who has read this far will recognise: digestion first, then energy, then mood, then the creeping feeling that her body had betrayed her again. It was the healing hierarchy in reverse. The downstream systems failing first as the upstream foundations eroded. When I ran her bloods, the data confirmed what the symptoms were telling us. On her stool test her zonulin was climbing. Her ferritin had dropped below thirty. Her B12 was drifting back toward the low end of the range. The systems had not failed. They had been left unsupported, and they were reverting.

Her body had not betrayed her. She had mistaken intervention for cure. She had confused feeling better with being finished.

This is the most common mistake I see in functional medicine. Not from practitioners, but from patients. Protocols work. Systems restore. Symptoms resolve. Then the patient assumes that the restoration is self-sustaining without any ongoing support. For some, it is. For many, it isn't, particularly those whose genetic vulnerabilities, environmental exposures, or lifestyle pressures remain. This chapter is about the difference between a protocol and a practice, and why the most important phase of recovery is the one that comes after the symptoms disappear.

Why Supplement Stacking Fails

Before I explain how to build a recovery plan that lasts, I need to address the approach that most people use instead, and why it fails.

Supplement stacking is the practice of adding interventions based on symptoms, recommendations, or trends without a systematic approach behind them. The patient reads that magnesium helps with anxiety, so they add magnesium. They hear that ashwagandha supports cortisol, so they add ashwagandha. They see that NAC is good for detoxification, so they add NAC. Within months they are taking fifteen to twenty supplements, spending hundreds of dollars a month, and have no idea which ones are working, which are redundant, and which may be actively interfering with each other.

Adding an iron supplement when the gut can't absorb it is waste. Adding a liver support when the gut is still producing the toxins that overwhelm the liver is premature. Adding a neurotransmitter precursor when the cofactors required to convert it are depleted is pointless.

Sequence matters more than substances. Alex is the clearest example: before he came to my clinic, a well-meaning practitioner had prescribed NAC for detoxification and 5-HTP for anxiety, both clinically valid, but without first addressing his Clostridia load and cofactor depletion, neither had any meaningful effect. The wrong supplement in a sensitised system doesn't just waste money. It can trigger a reaction that sets recovery back months and deepens the distrust that brought the patient to the clinic in the first place. This has been the argument of every chapter in this book, and it applies to the recovery plan itself.

The three-phase supplement philosophy I use in clinic is simple.

· Phase one: stabilise — calm the inflammation, repair the gut, address immediate deficiencies.

· Phase two: clear — remove pathogens, support detoxification, restore methylation.

· Phase three: optimise — support hormonal balance, add neurotransmitter precursors, build long-term resilience.

Each phase creates the conditions for the next. Skip a phase and the interventions in the subsequent phase either fail or produce unpredictable results.

There is also a concept I call protocol fatigue. It is the moment, usually around month three or four, when the patient looks at the number of supplements on their recovery plan and feels overwhelmed. The motivation that carried them through the first weeks fades. Compliance drops. They start skipping doses, then skipping days, then stopping entire categories of support. This is not a failure of willpower. It is a failure of communication. If the patient does not understand *why* each supplement is there, *how long* it needs to be taken, and *when* it can be removed, protocol fatigue is inevitable. The recovery plan must be built with an exit strategy for every intervention.

How a Recovery Plan Is Built

Every recovery plan in my clinic begins with data, not symptoms. The test results — blood panel, organic acids test, stool test, and, where relevant, hair tissue mineral analysis — provide the map. The symptoms provide the context. But the plan is built from the data, because the data reveals the upstream drivers that the symptoms cannot.

The four cases in this section illustrate the principle. Sarah's recovery plan began with gut repair because her data showed intestinal permeability and pathogen overgrowth driving autoimmune activation. James's plan began with Clostridia clearance because his OAT showed neurotoxins disrupting mitochondrial function. Emma's plan began with gut and mineral repletion because her data showed that thyroid autoimmunity was being sustained by intestinal permeability and cofactor depletion. Alex's plan began with blood sugar stabilisation and gut repair because his data showed Clostridia interference with neurotransmitter production alongside severe nutrient depletion.

Four different patients. Four different presentations. Four different starting points. But the same architecture: identify, address, build.

Identify the upstream driver from the data, address it first, and build the subsequent phases on the foundation that the first phase creates.

The plan itself is designed to evolve as the patient's biochemistry changes. Supplements that are critical in month one may be unnecessary by month four. Interventions that would have been premature at the start become appropriate once the upstream systems have stabilised.

Supplements Are Tools, Not Lifelines

Most supplements in a recovery plan are temporary. They are taken to create a biochemical change, to restore a depleted nutrient, support a compromised pathway, or clear a pathogenic load. Once the change has been achieved and confirmed by retesting, many of those supplements can be tapered and eventually removed.

This is counterintuitive for patients who have spent months feeling better on a supplement regimen. The assumption is that stopping the supplements will cause a return of symptoms. Sometimes it does, and that tells us the underlying capacity has not yet been fully restored and the support needs to continue. But more often, the body has rebuilt the capacity that was missing, and the supplement is no longer doing meaningful work. The only way to know is to test, taper, and observe.

There are exceptions — supplements that I find most patients benefit from on an ongoing or longer-term basis.

Activated B vitamins are the most significant. The body uses B vitamins as cofactors in virtually every biochemical pathway, and many patients, particularly those with MTHFR variants or methylation vulnerabilities, do measurably better when they maintain a baseline supply of methylated or activated B vitamins.

Probiotics are the second. The gut microbiome requires ongoing support, particularly in patients who have undergone antimicrobial treatment or who have limited dietary diversity. A quality spore-based probiotic and/or multi-strain formulation, taken consistently or pulsed through the plan, helps maintain the gut integrity that was rebuilt during the acute phase.

Detoxification support is the third. For patients with genetic vulnerabilities in Phase II detox pathways, or those with ongoing environmental exposures, periodic support with NAC, glutathione, or liver-specific herbs helps maintain the clearance capacity that was restored during treatment. This is typically pulsed rather than continuous, a few weeks on followed by a few weeks off.

In addition, a mineral formula of zinc, selenium, and key trace minerals, remains valuable for many patients whose dietary intake does not reliably meet optimal thresholds.

Beyond those, the goal is always to reduce the supplement load over time. Your body is designed to maintain its own biochemistry when the inputs are adequate and the systems are functioning. A recovery plan rebuilds the body's ability to function independently. Supplements speed up the process. They are not the process itself.

Retesting and Adjusting Based on Impact

The most important habit in long-term health management is periodic retesting. Not obsessive testing, not monthly panels driven by anxiety, but structured, purposeful retesting at intervals that match the biochemistry being addressed.

For acute interventions, gut repair, antimicrobial treatment, nutrient repletion, I recommend retesting at three months. For chronic issues, hormonal rebalancing, methylation, detoxification, six months is more appropriate. For ongoing monitoring, an annual review is the minimum: a blood panel at minimum, ideally with an organic acids test and stool test alongside it.

The retesting is about catching regression before it becomes symptomatic, not just confirming improvement. Biochemical changes often precede symptoms by weeks or months. A rising homocysteine level tells you that methylation is slipping before the fatigue and brain fog return. An elevation in zonulin tells you that gut permeability is increasing before the food sensitivities re-emerge. An upward trend in CRP tells you that inflammation is building before the joint pain or mood changes appear. Retesting allows you to intervene at the biochemical level rather than waiting for the clinical level, and that is the difference between prevention and reaction. The purpose of retesting is not to chase numbers. It is to catch drift before it becomes relapse.

Adjustment follows a simple decision framework. If the markers are improving and symptoms are resolving, stay the course and begin tapering supports as the data confirms restoration. If the markers have plateaued, improved but are not yet optimal, dig deeper. Look for missed drivers: environmental exposures, ongoing stress, sleep disruption, dietary lapses, or hidden infections that weren't addressed in the initial plan. If the markers are worsening despite compliance, pause and reassess. Something has changed, a new stressor, a new exposure, a system that wasn't adequately addressed, and the plan needs to adapt.

This is the principle that governs every recovery: adjustment is not failure. Adjustment is the strategy.

Measuring Progress: The Stability Score

Patients often ask me how to know whether they are truly getting better. Symptom tracking is useful but incomplete — symptoms fluctuate, and a bad day does not mean the plan is failing. Lab results are definitive but infrequent — you can't run a blood panel every week. What patients need is a practical, self-assessed metric that tracks the trend rather than the day.

I developed the Stability Score for this purpose. It is a zero-to-ten scale that measures predictability and resilience, not just symptom reduction.

A score of zero to three means crisis. Symptoms are unpredictable. Flares occur without clear triggers. Recovery from any stressor is slow and disproportionate. Life is organised around managing the illness. This is where most patients begin.

A score of four to six means improving but fragile. Good days are appearing, but setbacks are still common. Some triggers are identifiable, others are not. Progress feels real but inconsistent, and the fear of regression is constant.

A score of seven to eight means stable and predictable. Occasional flares still occur, but they are tied to identifiable triggers and the body recovers within a reasonable timeframe. The patient can plan their life around their health rather than organising their life around their illness. This is the target range within six to twelve months of beginning a structured recovery plan.

A score of nine to ten means resilient and optimised. The body responds predictably to all inputs, flares are rare and easily managed, and recovery is strong. The patient's focus has shifted from survival to performance and longevity. This is not the absence of all symptoms. It is the presence of a system that can handle the demands of life without collapsing.

Alex arrived at my clinic as a two — panic attacks dictating his days, grades collapsing, social life abandoned. By month three he had moved to a five:

good days appearing, but setbacks still common. By month five he was at eight — stable, predictable, and planning his future again. Emma followed a similar arc: a three at presentation, a six by month three as her thyroid markers stabilised, and an eight by month nine.

The Stability Score is assessed monthly, not daily, because daily variation obscures the trend. It is the metric that determines when a patient is ready to progress from one phase to the next, when supplements can be tapered, and when retesting is warranted. A plateau or regression in the Stability Score is the clearest signal that something in the plan needs to change.

Healing Is Not Linear

Every patient needs to hear this, and most need to hear it more than once: healing is not linear. There will be weeks where symptoms improve dramatically. There will be weeks where nothing seems to change. There will be weeks where symptoms temporarily worsen, particularly during die-off reactions when pathogens are being cleared, or during the early stages of dietary change when the body is adapting to a very different input.

Die-off, known clinically as a Herxheimer reaction, occurs when pathogenic organisms are being eliminated and they release toxins as they die. The symptoms can mimic the very condition being treated: digestive disruption, fatigue, headaches, body aches, skin changes, mood instability. Patients who are not warned about this often assume these symptoms are a sign the treatment is failing and they stop prematurely. Treatment is not failing. Instead, the body is clearing. Symptoms of die-off are temporary, typically lasting a few days to two weeks, and they resolve as the detoxification pathways process the load.

Alex experienced exactly this at week two of his Clostridia clearance. His anxiety briefly intensified, his sleep worsened, and he nearly stopped the protocol. Two weeks later, his panic attacks stopped entirely.

Progress is cumulative, not constant. The patient who feels only marginally better at week four may look at their data at month five and see markers that have shifted profoundly. The gap between how recovery feels and what recovery looks like on paper is one of the most important things a practitioner can help a patient understand.

The Practice, Not the Protocol

Kate made a mistake that was entirely understandable. She felt better. She assumed that meant she was finished. What she did not understand, and what I hadn't communicated clearly enough, was that the recovery plan had restored her capacity, but maintaining that capacity required ongoing attention to the fundamentals: diet, sleep, stress management, periodic testing, and a small number of foundational supplements tailored to her specific vulnerabilities.

This is the shift that separates a protocol from a practice. A protocol is a time-limited intervention designed to restore function. It has a beginning, a middle, and an end. A practice is the ongoing set of habits, inputs, and monitoring that maintains the function the protocol restored. The protocol is the intensive care unit. The practice is the lifestyle that keeps you out of it.

For most patients, the practice is a clean diet appropriate to their tolerances. Seven to eight hours of quality sleep. Regular movement. Stress awareness. An activated B vitamin and a probiotic most days. An annual set of blood work, and an organic acids test and stool test when warranted, to catch any drift before it becomes a problem. It is the willingness to adjust when the data or the symptoms suggest that something has shifted.

The four patients in this section each arrived at a different version of this practice.

Sarah's required ongoing attention to gut integrity and autoimmune triggers.

James's required sustained methylation support and mitochondrial maintenance.

Emma's required mineral monitoring and hormonal awareness through perimenopause.

Alex's required continued B6 and zinc supplementation to offset his pyrrole losses, and dietary habits that kept his blood sugar stable.

None of them are taking the full supplement plans they started with. All of them are maintaining the capacity those plans built.

This is what it means to move from crisis to resilience. The crisis is addressed by the protocol. The resilience is sustained by the practice. And the practice is guided by data, not fear, not habit, not guesswork, but the same testing, sequencing, and adjusting that resolved the crisis in the first place.

A protocol ends. A practice does not.

Systems restoration is now complete. Gut, biochemistry, hormones, and neurotransmitters have been addressed in sequence. A methodology for building, monitoring, and adjusting recovery plans has been laid out. What follows moves into territory that extends beyond systems restoration: environmental toxins and mould exposure, genetic variants that alter the recovery trajectory, and the biological architecture of longevity. The framework does not change. The investigation deepens.

If you want to see how this methodology translates into guided, step-by-step implementation, my Functional Medicine Solution Program applies the same framework described in this book in real time, with clinical structure and support:

functionalmedicinesolution.com

Protocol breakdowns, follow-up templates, and supplement duration guides are available at TheHealingHierarchy.com.

The protocol is never the endpoint. The data tells you when to adjust, when to hold, and when to let go.

Your workbook includes the Protocol vs. Practice Separator — a table that identifies which of your current supplements are time-limited protocols and which are ongoing practices.

PART VI

ADVANCED CASES

Chapter Fifteen

When Genetics Meet Depletion

Claire was thirty-eight when she sat in my clinic for the first time. She had conceived her first child easily at thirty-two. A healthy pregnancy, a healthy boy. But in the five years since, she had experienced three early miscarriages, each one more devastating than the last. Each loss carried its own grief, and the cumulative weight of three had left her physically and emotionally depleted. Her obstetrician had run the standard investigations: hormones, thyroid, pelvic ultrasound, chromosomal testing, nutrient screening. Everything came back within rangc.

"They keep telling me it's just bad luck," she said. "But I conceived my first baby so easily. What changed?"

From a conventional perspective, nothing had changed. Her labs were normal. Her anatomy was normal. Her chromosomes were normal. The working diagnosis was "unexplained recurrent pregnancy loss" — a clinical term that means *we have looked at everything we know how to look at, and we cannot find a reason.*

That isn't the same as there being no reason. It means the investigation was incomplete.

Claire's case is different from the four that preceded it. Sarah, James, Emma, and Alex each presented with symptoms that pointed clearly to a system in distress — digestive, energetic, hormonal, neurological. Claire's body was not producing obvious symptoms. It was failing under a specific, high-demand biological load: pregnancy. The reason it was failing is one of the most misunderstood concepts in functional medicine.

What MTHFR Actually Means

If you have spent any time in health communities online, you have almost certainly encountered MTHFR. It is one of the most discussed and least understood genetic variants in medicine. Some practitioners treat it as the root cause of everything. Some dismiss it as irrelevant. Both positions are wrong. Dr Ben Lynch's work, particularly *Dirty Genes*, did more than any other single contribution to bring methylation and genetic variants into mainstream clinical conversation. Where the field has sometimes oversimplified that work into "test MTHFR, take methylfolate," the clinical reality is more nuanced. Claire's case demonstrates why.

MTHFR stands for methylenetetrahydrofolate reductase. It is an enzyme that converts dietary folate into its active form — methylfolate - which the body uses to drive the methylation cycle. Methylation is not one reaction. It is a cascading series of chemical processes that affect DNA synthesis and repair, neurotransmitter production, hormone metabolism, detoxification, and immune regulation. When methylation works well, these processes run silently. When it doesn't, the effects are widespread but often invisible on standard testing.

The MTHFR gene has two well-studied variants: C677T and A1298C. A single copy of C677T reduces enzyme function by roughly twenty-five to thirty per cent. Two copies reduce it by forty to sixty per cent. The A1298C variant has a smaller effect individually, but when combined with C677T, a pattern called compound heterozygous, the cumulative reduction can reach fifty per cent.

But here is what most MTHFR discussions miss entirely:

The variant does not cause the problem. The variant reduces processing speed. Whether that reduced throughput becomes a clinical problem depends on how much demand the system is under and how well the cofactors are supplied.

A person with homozygous C677T who has excellent B12, folate, and B6 status, a healthy gut that absorbs nutrients efficiently, low inflammatory load, and manageable stress may methylate perfectly well for decades. The same person, under sustained stress, with gut dysfunction limiting absorption, with depleted cofactors and rising inflammation, will cross the threshold where reduced processing becomes functional failure. The gene did not change. The margin for error did.

Beyond MTHFR: The Methylation Network

MTHFR is only one enzyme in the methylation cycle. There are others that matter clinically, and Claire carried variants in several of them. Think of the methylation cycle as a relay — each enzyme passes the baton to the next, and a variant at any handover point slows the entire race.

MTR — methionine synthase — recycles homocysteine back into methionine, the precursor to SAMe, which is the body's primary methyl donor. A variant in MTR reduces the efficiency of this recycling. MTRR, methionine synthase reductase, regenerates the active form of vitamin B12 that MTR requires to function. A variant in MTRR means B12 is used up faster than it is regenerated. CBS — cystathionine beta-synthase — directs homocysteine down the transsulfuration pathway toward glutathione production, which governs detoxification and antioxidant defence.

Individually, each of these variants is common and usually silent. Roughly forty per cent of the population carries at least one MTHFR variant. Most will never know, because their system has enough capacity to compensate. But when multiple variants layer together, and that layering coincides with nutrient depletion, gut dysfunction, chronic stress, and inflammation. The combined effect creates a predictable bottleneck.

This is how methylation fails in clinical practice: not because of genes alone, but because demand exceeds capacity.

What Standard Testing Missed

Claire's GP had tested the things that GPs are trained to test. Serum B12 came back at 285 pmol/L, within the laboratory reference range of200 to 600. Serum folate was 18 nmol/L, within the range of 10 to 42. Her thyroid-stimulating hormone was 2.4 mIU/L, within the range of 0.4 to 4.0. By conventional standards, there was nothing to treat.

But functional testing tells a different story. Serum B12 measures total B12 in the blood, including inactive forms that the body can't use. Active B12, which measures only the biologically available form, came back at 42 pmol/L. The optimal threshold is above 80. Claire was not mildly low. She was severely depleted in the form of B12 that her methylation cycle actually depends on.

Serum folate looked adequate because it includes both natural folate and synthetic folic acid from fortified foods. For someone with MTHFR variants, synthetic folic acid can actually *block* folate receptors, occupying the binding site without being converted into the active methylfolate the body needs. Claire's folate was present in her blood. It wasn't reaching the pathway. This means that many women with MTHFR variants who are taking standard prenatal vitamins containing folic acid are not only receiving no benefit from the folate component, they may be actively blocking the receptor their body needs most. The solution is straightforward: replace synthetic folic acid with methylfolate, ideally under practitioner guidance, and the blockage resolves.

And her TSH of 2.4, while within the standard range, sits above the threshold of 2.0 that research associates with higher miscarriage risk. It was a thyroid that lacked optimal support for the demands of early pregnancy.

This is the recurring lesson of this book: normal does not mean optimal. In states of high biological demand — pregnancy, recovery, chronic illness — the gap between normal and optimal is where systems fail.

Claire's Data

The functional investigation revealed a system under compound pressure from multiple directions.

Blood panel. Homocysteine was 12.6 μmol/L, where optimal is 5 to 7. A direct marker of methylation bottleneck. Active B12 was 42 pmol/L, severely depleted. Ferritin was 28 ng/mL, where optimal for fertility is 50 to 150. Vitamin D was 52 nmol/L, below the functional optimal of 80. CRP was 2.8 mg/L, more than double the optimal threshold, chronic low-grade inflammation that mirrored what we saw in Sarah, James, and Alex.

Genetic testing. MTHFR C677T homozygous, two copies, roughly sixty to seventy per cent reduced enzyme activity. MTHFR A1298C wild type, no further reduction. MTR A2756G heterozygous, reduced homocysteine recycling. MTRR A66G homozygous, impaired B12 regeneration. CBS C699T heterozygous, variable glutathione production. This was not one variant. It was a network of processing bottlenecks that, under load, converged into a single clinical pattern: methylation failure.

Organic acids test. Methylmalonic acid was elevated. A functional marker confirming B12 deficiency at the tissue level, irrespective of what serum B12 showed. Uracil was elevated, confirming folate insufficiency in the pathway. Pyroglutamic acid was 38.5, where normal is below 28, indicating severe glutathione depletion and compromised detoxification capacity. Quinolinate was elevated, pointing to functional B6 deficiency.

Stool test. Calprotectin was 88, where normal is below 50, gut inflammation. Secretory IgA was low at 320, indicating impaired gut immune function. Lactobacillus and Bifidobacterium were depleted. Akkermansia, the gut barrier protector we discussed in Sarah's case, was absent. Beta-glucuronidase was elevated, impairing the clearance of used hormones including oestrogen and progesterone.

Claire's day-21 progesterone was 26 nmol/L, below the 30 nmol/L threshold for healthy luteal support. This was a downstream consequence of impaired hormone clearance and depleted cofactors. The same pattern Emma demonstrated with her thyroid: the hormone was failing because everything upstream of it was compromised.

The Gut–Methylation Connection

Claire's gut dysfunction was not incidental. It was the accelerant.

Methylation depends on a continuous supply of folate, B12, B6, amino acids, choline, and betaine. Every one of those nutrients must be absorbed through the gut lining. When the gut is inflamed, when the microbial balance is disrupted, when the immune barrier is compromised, absorption falls, and the methylation cycle, which was already running at reduced speed due to Claire's genetic variants, lost even more capacity.

This created a vicious cycle. Impaired methylation reduces the body's ability to maintain the gut lining, produce adequate stomach acid, and regulate the immune response in the gut. Which further impairs absorption and further depletes the cofactors that methylation requires. The system spirals. Each pregnancy attempt placed additional demand on a cycle that was already in deficit, and each loss deepened the depletion.

Her first pregnancy succeeded because, at thirty-two, her reserves were still adequate. She had lower stress, better sleep, stronger absorption, and fewer competing physiological demands. Over the following five years, through post-partum recovery, cumulative stress, three pregnancy losses and the grief that accompanied them, and progressive gut dysfunction. Her buffer eroded until it could no longer sustain the biochemical demands of early pregnancy.

Her genes remained the same. Her capacity had shifted.

Restoring Capacity

The intervention followed the same sequencing principles that governed every case in this book, but with a specific focus on methylation bypass and cofactor restoration.

The first and most urgent step was to clear the blocker. Synthetic folic acid was eliminated from Claire's diet entirely. This meant eliminating fortified breads, cereals, and the standard prenatal vitamin she had been taking. For someone with her MTHFR profile, synthetic folic acid was not merely unhelpful. It was actively competing with the methylfolate her body needed.

Phase one — restore absorption. This addressed gut repair and nutrient absorption in parallel. The same principles from Sarah's chapter applied: repair the gut lining, rebalance the microbiome, reduce inflammation, and restore the immune barrier. Without this foundation, the methylation-specific interventions that followed would have been absorbed poorly and converted inefficiently.

Phase two — bypass the bottleneck. This targeted the methylation bottleneck directly. Methylfolate replaced synthetic folic acid, bypassing the MTHFR enzyme entirely and delivering the active form directly. Methylcobalamin and hydroxocobalamin provided active B12 to support the MTR and MTRR pathways. P-5-P, active vitamin B6, addressed the functional B6 deficiency confirmed on her OAT. Betaine supported an alternative methylation pathway that doesn't depend on MTHFR at all.

Phase three — rebuild the shield. NAC, glycine, and alpha-lipoic acid supported the transsulfuration pathway that Claire's CBS variant had made less efficient. Pyroglutamic acid at 38.5 told us her glutathione was severely depleted. This is the same marker we tracked in Alex's case, and the same restoration pathway.

Phase four — optimise for conception. Selenium for thyroid hormone conversion. TSH monitoring every six to eight weeks, targeting below 2.0. Omega-3 fatty acids for inflammation and hormonal balance. CoQ10 for mitochondrial support and egg quality. And progesterone monitoring to confirm that the luteal phase was strengthening as the upstream systems restored.

Throughout, stress reduction was critical — magnesium, L-theanine, ashwagandha, sleep hygiene, breathwork. Not as luxuries, as clinical interventions. Chronic stress depletes methylation cofactors directly, raises cortisol, and impairs implantation. For Claire, every stressor was a withdrawal from an account that was already overdrawn.

The Outcome

At eight months, Claire's follow-up data told the story. Homocysteine had normalised from 12.6 to 6.2 μmol/L. Active B12 had risen from 42 to 128 pmol/L. Ferritin had restored to 92 ng/mL. Vitamin D reached 135 nmol/L. CRP dropped to 0.6 mg/L. TSH settled at 1.4 mIU/L. Day-21 progesterone rose to 42 nmol/L, a healthy luteal phase. Pyroglutamic acid normalised, confirming glutathione restoration. Her gut markers, calprotectin, secretory IgA, bacterial diversity, had all returned to optimal ranges.

Claire conceived naturally at month nine.

She carried to term. A healthy pregnancy. A healthy baby. After three losses and five years of being told nothing was wrong, she held a child that her biochemistry had finally been able to support. And in the years that followed, two more pregnancies — both carried to term, both healthy deliveries.

"I don't understand why nobody tested any of this before. Three miscarriages, and the answer was there the whole time."

Genes Are Instructions, Not Outcomes

Claire's case teaches the principle that sits at the centre of every advanced case in this section of the book: genetics reveal where the weaker pathways are, but they don't have to define the outcome. The outcome is determined by whether the system has the ability to compensate, and that ability depends on cofactor supply, gut function, inflammatory load, and physiological demand.

This is why genetic testing alone is insufficient. Knowing that a patient carries MTHFR variants tells you that their folate conversion is slower than average. It doesn't tell you whether their folate levels are adequate, whether their B12 is sufficient, whether their gut can absorb the nutrients they need, or whether their methylation is functionally impaired. For that, you need the organic acids test, the blood panel, and the stool test. The genes provide the context. The functional tests provide the data.

The mistake many practitioners make, and many patients make after discovering their MTHFR status online, is to treat the gene variant directly with methylfolate and methyl-B12 without assessing the system those nutrients enter. If the gut is inflamed and absorption is poor, even methylfolate is less effective, which is why gut repair runs in parallel, not after. If B6 is depleted, the methylation cycle stalls irrespective of folate status. If glutathione is depleted, the detoxification pathway that depends on methylation's output is compromised. The gene is one variable in a multi-variable system. Treating it in isolation is the same error as treating any single downstream symptom without addressing what drives it.

When foundational pathways lose function, the most demanding systems fail first. For Claire, the most demanding system was pregnancy. For another patient with the same genetic profile, it might be mood, or energy, or immune function. The genetics determine where the system is most vulnerable. The upstream investigation determines why it is failing now.

For Claire, the miscarriages carried their own grief, being told nothing was wrong, three times, left a different kind of wound.

Claire's case is the first in this section to introduce genetic vulnerability as a clinical variable. The next chapter introduces Marcus, whose systems appeared to be failing for the same reasons we have seen throughout this book: gut dysfunction, nutrient depletion, and inflammation, but whose recovery stalled until we identified the environmental exposure that was sustaining the entire pattern.

Same framework. Deeper investigation.

CLAIRE Fertility & Methylation (9 months to conception)

MARKER	BEFORE		AFTER
Homocysteine	12.6 µmol/L	→	6.2 µmol/L
Active B12	42 pmol/L	→	580 pmol/L
Folate	Low	→	Optimised
MTHFR C677T	Identified	→	Supported
Pyroglutamic Acid	Elevated	→	Normalised
TSH	Borderline	→	Optimised

Conceived naturally at month 9 after three prior miscarriages.

Claire's methylation protocol is available at TheHealingHierarchy.com.

Her genes remained the same. Her body, once supported, was more than capable.

Chapter Sixteen

When the Gut Is Not the Problem

Marcus was forty-five, a software engineer, and he had been living on twelve foods for three years. Not by choice. By elimination. Three years of twelve foods had contracted his world. No restaurants, no shared meals, no spontaneity around food. Every time he tried to expand his diet, his body punished him — bloating within thirty minutes, brain fog by the afternoon, anxiety after meals that had no psychological cause. He had seen four practitioners, completed two antimicrobial gut protocols, tried a low-FODMAP diet, a candida protocol, and a comprehensive elimination diet. Each time, he improved for a few weeks. And each time, the symptoms returned.

"I've been told my gut is the problem," he said at our first appointment. "But every time we treat my gut, it comes back. I'm starting to think this is just how I am now."

It wasn't how he was. His gut wasn't the problem. His gut was where the problem was showing up. The actual driver was sitting downstream, in the detoxification pathways that were supposed to process what his gut absorbed, and until those pathways were addressed, every gut protocol he tried would produce the same pattern: temporary relief followed by predictable relapse.

Marcus's case is the second in this section to demonstrate that some patients require investigation beyond the standard systems restoration approach. Claire's system was failing because genetic methylation variants had created a processing bottleneck under load. Marcus's system was failing because genetic detoxification variants had created a processing bottleneck under toxic load. In both cases, the standard gut chapter — Chapter 10 — would have been insufficient. In both cases, the upstream driver was not in the gut itself but in the body's capacity to handle what the gut was producing.

The Pattern That Reveals the Problem

Before I looked at any of Marcus's test results, his food reactivity pattern told me where to investigate.

He reacted to sulfur foods: eggs, cruciferous vegetables, garlic, onions. He reacted to histamine foods: aged cheese, wine, fermented foods, leftovers. He reacted to phenol foods: berries, coffee, dark chocolate. And glutamine, the amino acid most commonly recommended for gut repair, made him worse. Glutamine converts to glutamate in the body, an excitatory neurotransmitter. In a patient with a slow COMT variant who already clears excitatory compounds poorly, supplemental glutamine can amplify anxiety, insomnia, and neurological reactivity rather than heal the gut.

Each of these categories maps to a specific detoxification pathway. Sulfur compounds are processed by the sulfation pathway, which depends on the SULT1A1 enzyme. Histamine is broken down by the DAO enzyme and cleared through methylation. Phenols are processed through phase one detoxification, which depends on the CYP1A2 enzyme. When a patient reacts to *all three categories at once,* it is not a food problem. It is a processing problem. The body can't clear what it is absorbing.

This pattern is one of the most commonly misdiagnosed presentations in functional medicine. Practitioners see the food reactions and focus on the gut. They run a stool test, find some dysbiosis, prescribe antimicrobials, and the patient improves, because reducing the microbial load temporarily reduces the toxic output that the detox pathways cannot handle. But the detox pathways have not been restored. So the microbial load rebuilds, the toxic output rises, and the food reactions return. The practitioner increases the antimicrobial dose, the patient restricts their diet further, and the cycle repeats. I have seen patients arrive at my clinic on three or four foods, having been through multiple rounds of gut treatment, when the gut was never the primary problem.

How Marcus Got Here

Three years before I saw him, Marcus had contracted severe food poisoning while travelling overseas. He was hospitalised briefly and treated with two rounds of broad-spectrum antibiotics. The antibiotics saved him from the acute infection. They also devastated his gut microbiome.

Within months, he developed chronic bloating, alternating constipation and diarrhoea, and an expanding list of food sensitivities. His GP diagnosed irritable bowel syndrome. A naturopath diagnosed candida overgrowth. A functional medicine practitioner diagnosed SIBO and prescribed herbal antimicrobials. Each diagnosis contained a piece of the truth, but none of them identified the complete pattern.

The antibiotics had eliminated the beneficial bacteria that normally keep opportunistic organisms in check. In the absence of that microbial balance, methane-producing organisms colonised his small intestine, creating methane-dominant SIBO. Clostridia species overgrew, producing neurotoxins. Fungal organisms expanded, producing their own toxic metabolites. His gut became a factory of compounds that his body was supposed to process and eliminate. But his body couldn't keep up.

Marcus's Data

The investigation revealed why his body couldn't keep up.

SIBO breath test. Methane was 48 parts per million, where positive is above 10. This confirmed methane-dominant SIBO — Methanobrevibacter smithii colonising the small intestine, causing bloating, constipation, and producing neurotoxic byproducts.

Organic acids test. HPHPA, the Clostridia marker we tracked in James's and Alex's cases, was 18.5, where normal is below 4.5. Severely elevated. Tricarballylic acid, a marker of fungal overgrowth, was 8.2, where normal is below 2.5. Pyroglutamic acid was 48.5, where normal is below 28. The highest glutathione depletion of any case in this book, including Alex's 41.5. His body's master detoxification molecule was critically exhausted — sulfate was low, confirming impaired sulfation, and xanthurenate was elevated, confirming functional B6 deficiency.

Genetic testing. This is where the picture crystallised. SULT1A1 homozygous, impaired sulfation, explaining his inability to process sulfur compounds. COMT slow variant, slow clearance of dopamine and catecholamines, explaining his heightened sensitivity to stimulatory compounds and his anxiety after meals. CYP1A2 slow variant, slow phase one detoxification, explaining why caffeine and phenol compounds lingered in his system. MTHFR A1298C homozygous, reduced methylation capacity, impairing detox and neurotransmitter recycling. GSTM1 deletion. A complete absence of the glutathione S-transferase M1 enzyme, meaning one of the major pathways for conjugating toxins with glutathione was simply missing.

Individually, each of these variants is manageable. Millions of people carry them without symptoms. But layered together, under the sustained toxic load from SIBO, Clostridia, and fungal overgrowth, they created a processing bottleneck that no amount of gut treatment alone could resolve.

Blood panel. Plasma histamine was 18.5, where normal is below 10, nearly double. DAO activity was low, confirming that the enzyme responsible for breaking down histamine in the gut was overwhelmed. Copper was elevated. Zinc was low. B6 was low. Magnesium was low.

Stool test. And here is the detail that makes this case distinctive: Marcus's GI-MAP was largely unremarkable. No major pathogens. No parasites. Mild imbalance only. If a practitioner had relied on the stool test alone, as many do, they would have concluded that his gut was essentially normal and looked elsewhere. The stool test missed the problem because the problem was not in the gut. It was in the body's ability to process what the gut was producing.

Why Gut Protocols Keep Failing

The logic of Marcus's repeated treatment failures was now visible.

His SIBO and fungal overgrowth were producing toxic byproducts — phenols, amines, sulfur compounds, neurotoxins. His genetic detox variants limited how fast he could clear those compounds. The toxins accumulated, his gut became inflamed, and food sensitivities expanded. A practitioner prescribed antimicrobials, which temporarily reduced the microbial load. Symptoms improved. But the detox pathways were still blocked. The microbial load rebuilt. The toxins accumulated again. Symptoms returned.

It is like bailing water from a boat without repairing the hull. You can reduce the water level temporarily, but until you fix the structural breach, the boat keeps flooding.

This is the clinical principle Marcus's case teaches: when gut protocols repeatedly fail, the problem is often metabolic, not microbial. The gut is producing more than the body can process. Restore the processing capacity, and the gut protocols that previously failed begin to hold.

Restoring Processing Function

The intervention ran simultaneously on two tracks: eradicate the microbial overgrowth, and restore the detoxification pathways that had been overwhelmed by it.

Phase 1 — eradicate and restore motility. Methane-targeted herbal antimicrobials, allicin, neem, berberine, and oregano oil on rotation, addressed the SIBO directly. Prokinetic support with ginger root extract and partially hydrolysed guar gum restored gut motility, which is essential for preventing SIBO relapse. Motility is the mechanism that sweeps bacteria out of the small intestine between meals. When motility fails, often after food poisoning or gastroenteritis, bacteria accumulate in territory they shouldn't occupy. Restoring motility is not supplementary to SIBO treatment. It is the reason SIBO does not return.

Phase 2 — reduce the toxic load. A temporary low-histamine, low-sulfur, low-phenol diet removed the dietary inputs that Marcus's detox pathways could not process. This was not a permanent dietary restriction. It was a strategic pause, reducing the incoming load while the pathways were being rebuilt, so the system wasn't overwhelmed from both directions at once.

Phase 3 — rebuild detox capacity. Glycine was the first glutathione precursor introduced. A non-sulfur amino acid that Marcus could tolerate even with his SULT1A1 variant. NAC was added cautiously at week nine and titrated slowly, because sulfur-containing compounds had to be introduced at a pace his sulfation pathway could manage. P-5-P, active vitamin B6, supported the sulfation pathway directly as a SULT1A1 cofactor. Molybdenum supported sulfite oxidase, helping his body process the sulfur compounds that had been accumulating. DAO enzyme taken before meals helped break down histamine while his own body's ability to process rebuilt. Quercetin stabilised mast cells, reducing the histamine release that had been driving much of his neurological reactivity.

Phase 4 — gentle methylation. Because Marcus carried COMT slow and MTHFR A1298C homozygous, standard methylation support, methylfolate and methyl-B12, risked over-methylating his already slow COMT pathway, potentially worsening his anxiety. Instead, folinic acid replaced methylfolate, and hydroxocobalamin replaced methyl-B12. Both are gentler forms that support methylation without the stimulatory effect of their methyl counterparts. This is the clinical nuance that Claire's chapter introduced: "the form of the supplement matters as much as the nutrient itself, and the patient's genetics, symptoms, and tolerance determine which form is appropriate.

Phase 5 — food reintroduction. Beginning at month seven, with detox pathways restored and microbial overgrowth cleared, foods were reintroduced in the order of the pathways they challenged. Sulfur foods first, eggs, garlic, onions, cruciferous vegetables, one at a time, tracking reactions. Histamine foods second, fermented foods, aged cheese, wine. Phenol foods third, berries, coffee, dark chocolate. The reintroduction was systematic and data-informed. If a food triggered a reaction, it was pulled back and the supporting protocol was continued for another four weeks before retrying.

The Outcome

Within weeks of beginning the combined protocol, Marcus's bloating reduced dramatically. His bowel habits stabilised. The brain fog and post-meal anxiety diminished.

At month four, retesting confirmed the shift. SIBO breath test: methane normalised. OAT: HPHPA dropped to 2.8, Clostridia cleared. Tricarballylic acid normalised, fungal overgrowth resolved. Pyroglutamic acid came down to 22.5 signaling that glutathione was restored. Sulfate normalised. B6 normalised. Plasma histamine dropped from 18.5 to 6.8. DAO activity improved.

By month ten, Marcus was eating eggs, garlic, fermented foods, coffee, dark chocolate, and wine. Foods he had not been able to touch in three years. His diet had expanded from twelve foods to a normal, varied intake. His ten-month retest confirmed the restoration was holding: pyroglutamic acid stable, histamine within range, SIBO breath test clear.

"I'm eating things I haven't been able to touch in years," he said at his final follow-up. "And I'm not reacting. It's not that I'm managing symptoms anymore — I just don't have them."

MARCUS — Food Reactivity & Detox Restoration (6 months)

MARKER	BEFORE		AFTER
Pyroglutamic Acid	Elevated	→	Normalised
Glutathione	Depleted	→	Restored
Oxalate Markers	Elevated	→	Normalised
Clostridia Markers	Elevated	→	Cleared
Food Tolerance	12 foods only	→	Varied diet

Expanded from 12 foods to a varied diet. Reactivity resolved.

From The Healing Hierarchy by Jarrod Cooper - ND

Tolerance Is the Goal

Marcus's case redefines what recovery looks like for patients with complex food sensitivities. The goal isn't a longer list of safe foods managed by avoidance. It's tolerance. The ability to eat a varied diet without the body reacting to normal dietary compounds.

Tolerance is not a dietary achievement. It is a metabolic one. It means the detoxification pathways can process what the gut absorbs. It means the gut isn't producing more than the body can handle. It means the system has capacity.

This is where Marcus's case connects to Claire's. Both patients carried genetic variants that reduced specific biochemical processing. Both were told their problem was elsewhere — Claire in her reproductive system, Marcus in his gut. Both had received treatments that addressed the wrong level of the system. Both recovered when the actual bottleneck was identified and restored. For Marcus, one distinction matters for the long term: his GSTM1 deletion means one of his major glutathione conjugation pathways is permanently absent. It can't be repaired. It can be supplemented. Consistent glutathione precursor support - glycine, NAC, and alpha-lipoic acid - is a permanent maintenance requirement for him.

The pattern also connects backward to the standard cases. Sarah's autoimmunity was driven by her gut. James's fatigue was driven by Clostridia toxicity and mitochondrial disruption. Emma's thyroid was driven by cofactor depletion and gut permeability. Alex's anxiety was driven by neurotransmitter precursor failure. Claire's pregnancy losses were driven by methylation failure under genetic load. And Marcus's food intolerances were driven by detox bottlenecks under microbial load.

Six patients. Six different presentations. The same architecture: identify the upstream driver, address it in sequence, and monitor the restoration with data.

When gut protocols repeatedly fail, stop treating the gut harder. Ask what the gut is producing that the body can't process. Ask what processing pathways are compromised. Ask what genetic, nutritional, or environmental factors are limiting processing capacity. The answer is rarely more antimicrobials. The answer is almost always a system that hasn't been fully investigated.

The next chapter introduces the most complex environmental case in this book — Rachel, whose illness was sustained not by anything happening inside her body, but by the building she was living in.

Same framework. New variable: the environment.

Chapter Seventeen

When the Building Is the Problem

Rachel was thirty-five when she moved her family into a beautiful new rental. Within six months, her health collapsed. Sleep shattered. Panic attacks began on a daily basis, unprovoked, with no psychological trigger. Brain fog so dense she couldn't follow conversations. Energy so depleted she could barely get her children to school. Her digestion deteriorated. Her menstrual cycle stopped entirely. She went from a healthy, functioning mother of two to a woman who could not recognise her own body.

She saw her GP, who tested her thyroid and iron levels and found nothing abnormal. She saw a psychologist, who diagnosed generalised anxiety. She tried an elimination diet, which helped marginally. She tried supplements recommended online, magnesium, B vitamins, adaptogens, and felt no different. By month four, her children were showing signs of immune stress: recurrent infections, dark circles under their eyes, irritability that was out of character.

That's when Rachel realised the problem was bigger than just her. When the whole family is sick, the problem is rarely inside any one person's body. It is in the environment they share.

Before she came to me, Rachel had already been through the system. Her GP told her she had a case of 'motheritis' essentially, that being a tired mum was the diagnosis. A functional medicine doctor told her she had chronic fatigue. Neither looked beyond her body for the cause.

When Rachel came to me, the pattern was the first thing I noticed. Same house, same timeline, whole family declining. Before I ran a single test, I asked her about her home. When had they moved in? Had there been any water damage? What kind of ventilation did the property have?

I ordered a mycotoxin test. The results confirmed significant mould exposure. I referred her to a building biologist to inspect the property. They found extremely high mould levels in the air conditioning system and significant contamination in the roof space from a prior water leak. The system had been circulating mould spores through the house every time it ran. When they pulled back carpets and inspected soft furnishings, they found visible mould growth on clothing, bedding, and furniture.

Rachel was not losing her mind. She was being poisoned. And no amount of gut repair, methylation support, or stress management would have resolved her symptoms while she remained in that building.

What Mould Illness Actually Is

Mould illness — formally known as Chronic Inflammatory Response Syndrome, or CIRS, is not an allergy. It is a systemic inflammatory condition triggered by exposure to biotoxins, primarily mycotoxins produced by certain mould species. The distinction matters because allergies produce a localised immune response such as sneezing, watery eyes, a runny nose. CIRS produces a *whole-body* inflammatory cascade that can affect virtually every system: neurological, hormonal, immunological, digestive, and cardiovascular.

The clinical framework for understanding mould illness owes much to Dr Ritchie Shoemaker, whose research over two decades identified the biotoxin pathway, the role of HLA gene susceptibility, and the specific inflammatory markers, C4a, TGF-β1, MSH, and VIP, that distinguish

CIRS from the conditions it mimics. His work gave clinicians a testable, measurable map of what had previously been dismissed as psychosomatic. Where the field has continued to evolve is in the integration of mould illness within a broader systems framework — recognising that CIRS rarely exists in isolation, and that the gut dysfunction, methylation impairment, and hormonal disruption it produces must be addressed in sequence alongside the biotoxin clearance itself. Rachel's case demonstrates both Shoemaker's foundational insight and the layered clinical reality that follows from it.

Most people who are exposed to indoor mould will experience some degree of irritation and, upon leaving the environment, recover. But roughly twenty-four per cent of the population carries HLA gene variants that make them highly susceptible to biotoxins. In these individuals, the immune system can't efficiently recognise and clear mycotoxins. The toxins remain in circulation, triggering a chronic inflammatory loop that persists even after the exposure ends. The immune system doesn't turn off because it can't identify the toxin as cleared.

This is the genetic trap of CIRS. It is not that these individuals are weaker. It is that their immune surveillance system has a blind spot for a specific category of toxin. And when that blind spot meets sustained environmental exposure, the result is a multi-system collapse that mimics, and is frequently misdiagnosed as, anxiety, chronic fatigue syndrome, fibromyalgia, or autoimmune disease.

Rachel's Data

The functional investigation confirmed what the building inspection had revealed.

Genetic testing. HLA-DR/DQ testing confirmed a mould-susceptible haplotype. Rachel's immune system was genetically unable to clear mycotoxins efficiently. This explained why she was the sickest member of the household — same exposure, different genetic capacity to process it.

Urinary mycotoxins. Ochratoxin A was 12.5 ng/mg creatinine, where normal is below 1.8, seven times the upper limit. Gliotoxin was 0.85, where normal is below 0.20, four times elevated. Citrinin was 2.4, where normal is below 0.50, five times elevated. Her urine was saturated with mould toxins, evidence of both chronic exposure and impaired clearance.

CIRS biomarkers. C4a, a marker of innate immune activation, was 18,500 ng/mL, where normal is below 2,830. Six times the upper limit. Her immune system was in sustained overdrive. MMP-9 was 1,250, where normal is below 332, indicating vascular inflammation and blood-brain barrier permeability, which explained the severity of her brain fog. TGF-β1 was elevated at 5,800, where normal is below 2,380, indicating autoimmune and fibrosis risk.

Two markers told the deeper story. MSH — melanocyte-stimulating hormone, was critically low at 12, where normal is 35 to 81. MSH is produced by the hypothalamus and regulates sleep, hormone production, mood, and immune function. When MSH is suppressed by mycotoxins, every system it governs fails simultaneously. This single marker explained Rachel's insomnia, her lost menstrual cycle, her anxiety, and her immune dysfunction. VIP, vasoactive intestinal peptide, was low at 18, where normal is 23 to 63, explaining her gastrointestinal deterioration. These are the markers that conventional medicine does not test for, and without them, Rachel's presentation looks like anxiety, chronic fatigue, and hormonal dysfunction rather than what it actually was: environmental poisoning.

MARCoNS. Nasal culture was positive for Multiple Antibiotic Resistant Coagulase Negative Staphylococci. A type of antibiotic-resistant bacteria that forms protective biofilms in the nasal passages of mould-affected patients. In plain terms, Rachel's sinuses had been colonised by bacteria that produce their own neurotoxins and keep the inflammatory cascade active long after the original exposure. MARCoNS acts as a toxin amplifier, even after a patient leaves the mouldy environment, the nasal colonisation continues to drive the inflammatory response. It is one of the reasons patients with CIRS do not recover simply by leaving the building.

Gut and organic acids. GI-MAP showed severe Candida overgrowth at 5.2×10^7 CFU/g, where normal is below 1×10^6. OAT showed elevated Aspergillus markers. The mould exposure had seeded systemic fungal overgrowth in her gut. A secondary infection maintaining the inflammatory load from the inside even as the external exposure was being addressed.

You Cannot Detox Your Way Out of a Toxic Environment

This is the most important principle in environmental medicine, and it is the one most commonly violated: you can't supplement, bind, or protocol your way to health while the exposure continues. Every binder you take mobilises toxins. If you are still inhaling mould spores eight hours a night, the mobilised toxins are replaced faster than they are eliminated. The result is not recovery. It is redistribution, moving toxins around the body without reducing the total load.

Rachel had tried detox supplements before she came to me. They made her worse. This is the classic pattern in CIRS: aggressive detoxification without removal of the exposure produces a crash, not a clearing. The patient feels sicker, assumes the supplements are wrong, and stops. The supplements were not wrong. The sequence was.

The first step in mould illness is always the same, and it is non-negotiable: remove the exposure. Leave the building or remediate it thoroughly with professional help. For Rachel, this meant breaking the lease, moving to temporary housing, and discarding soft furnishings, clothing, bedding, and porous items that had absorbed mycotoxins. She lost belongings. She was heartbroken. But she finally had an answer.

Sequenced Recovery

With the exposure removed, the intervention followed a precise sequence.

Phase 1 — eradicate MARCoNS. MARCoNS had to be cleared first because it acts as a persistent driver of the inflammatory cascade. BEG nasal spray, a compounded prescription of Bactroban, EDTA, and Gentamicin, was administered twice daily for eight weeks to break down the biofilm and eliminate the antibiotic-resistant bacteria. Retest at week eight: MARCoNS negative.

Phase 2 — bind and eliminate mycotoxins. Natural binders were introduced from week one, running concurrently with the MARCoNS treatment. Activated charcoal, modified citrus pectin, and fulvic and humic acid-based mineral binders were rotated throughout the day, taken away from food and supplements to avoid nutrient depletion. Rachel experienced mild detox symptoms — fatigue, headaches, in the first week as toxins mobilised. They passed within days. Urinary mycotoxin levels dropped steadily without the need for pharmaceutical binders.

Phase 3 — clear systemic fungal overgrowth. Herbal antifungals, caprylic acid, oregano oil, and berberine, addressed the Candida and Aspergillus overgrowth that the mould exposure had seeded in her gut. Spore-based and multi-strain probiotics supported microbial rebalancing. This phase ran for twelve weeks alongside the binding protocol.

Phase 4 — restore detox capacity. Once binding was underway and the microbial load was reducing, glutathione support was introduced. Liposomal glutathione, NAC, glycine, and alpha-lipoic acid. The same glutathione restoration pathway used in Marcus's and Alex's cases, adapted here for a patient whose glutathione depletion was driven by mycotoxin load rather than genetic bottleneck or nutrient depletion.

Phase 5 — restore the hypothalamus. At month ten, with CIRS biomarkers improving and mycotoxin levels declining, VIP nasal spray was introduced under physician supervision. VIP, vasoactive intestinal peptide, is one of the final interventions in CIRS recovery because it addresses the hypothalamic suppression that drives the hormonal, sleep, and immune dysfunction. It isn't introduced early because it is ineffective while the inflammatory drivers are still active. Sequence, as always, determines efficacy.

Phase 6 — immune rebalancing. Omega-3 fatty acids, curcumin, vitamin D optimisation, and a low-amylose diet supported the transition from inflammatory crisis to immune restoration. This phase ran alongside phases four and five and continued beyond the formal treatment period as the foundation of Rachel's ongoing practice.

The Outcome

Rachel's recovery took fourteen months. The longest of any case in this book. CIRS does not resolve quickly, because the inflammatory cascade has penetrated multiple regulatory systems and each must be restored in sequence.

By month six, her mycotoxin levels had dropped significantly. MARCoNS was cleared. C4a had fallen from 18,500 to 4,200. Brain fog was lifting. Sleep was improving. By month ten, her energy had returned. CRP dropped to 0.5 mg/L. Candida was cleared. Aspergillus markers normalised. At month twelve, her menstrual cycle returned. The clearest sign that her hypothalamic function was restoring. By month fourteen, MSH had risen to 38, VIP had normalised, and her mycotoxin levels were undetectable.

Rachel got her life back. Her children's health normalised within weeks of leaving the house. Their immune systems, unburdened by genetic susceptibility, cleared the toxins on their own once the exposure stopped. Within a month, the dark circles were gone, the infections stopped, and the irritability that had worried Rachel almost as much as her own symptoms disappeared entirely.

Fourteen months is a long time to hold a household together while rebuilding your own biology. Rachel did it because she finally understood what was happening, and because, for the first time, the intervention matched the cause.

"I thought I was going crazy," she said. "Every doctor I saw treated me like it was in my head. It wasn't in my head. It was in my house."

When to Suspect the Environment

Rachel's case teaches the principle that governs this entire section of the book: when the standard framework has been applied correctly and the patient is not recovering, the investigation must expand beyond the body. The environment is the variable that functional medicine most often overlooks.

There are clinical signs that point toward environmental exposure as a driver. Multi-system symptoms that don't cluster around a single organ system — fatigue *plus* brain fog *plus* anxiety *plus* gut dysfunction *plus* hormonal disruption, are characteristic of CIRS. Symptoms that worsen in certain buildings and improve when the patient travels or stays elsewhere. Family members who are also unwell. A history of water damage, visible mould, or musty odours in the home or workplace. And CIRS-specific biomarkers: elevated C4a, elevated MMP-9, low MSH, low VIP.

The critical lesson is this: if you are following the right protocols, doing the foundational work, and still not responding, or responding temporarily and relapsing, ask about your environment. Ask about your home. Ask about your workplace. Ask about water damage. The answer may not be inside your body. It may be in the building you return to every night.

Seven patients across seven chapters. Sarah's gut. James's mitochondria. Emma's thyroid. Alex's neurotransmitters. Claire's methylation. Marcus's detox pathways. Rachel's environment. Each case extended the investigation one layer further. Each demonstrated that the same architecture, test, sequence, restore, monitor, applies regardless of where the driver is found. Claire's methylation variants, Marcus's detox variants, and Rachel's HLA profile each represent a different category of genetic susceptibility, but the principle is identical: genes determine vulnerability, environment and load determine whether that vulnerability becomes illness.

The advanced cases are now complete. What follows is the final dimension of this framework. Removing what harms the body is only half the work. The final section asks a different question: once the system is restored, how do you build a body that ages differently? That is where biological age, cellular resilience, and the longevity framework begin.

You can't heal in a toxic environment. But once the environment is clean, the body knows what to do.

RACHEL — Mould Illness & CIRS Recovery (14 months)

MARKER	BEFORE		AFTER
Mycotoxins (Ochratoxin A)	Elevated	→	Cleared
Mycotoxins (Gliotoxin)	Elevated	→	Cleared
MARCoNS Nasal Culture	Positive	→	Cleared
C4a	Elevated	→	Normalised
TGF-β1	Elevated	→	Normalised
VCS (Visual Contrast)	Failed	→	Passed
MMP-9	Elevated	→	Normalised

Full CIRS recovery after remediation + sequenced protocol.

Rachel's mould recovery protocol is available at TheHealingHierarchy.com.

PART VII

LONGEVITY

Chapter Eighteen

The Longevity Question

Michael was fifty-two and, by every standard measure, healthy. No diagnosis. No medication. No symptoms that would send him to a doctor. He exercised regularly, ate well, slept reasonably, and ran a successful consulting business. His GP had told him his bloods were "normal" at his last check-up. There was nothing wrong with Michael.

But something had shifted. Recovery from training was slower than it had been three years ago. His focus drifted in the afternoons, his energy, once reliable, now came in waves, and his libido had declined. None of it was dramatic. But he had started noticing that he no longer bounced back the way he used to, and he could not keep putting it down to just another "busy week." He was not sick. He wasn't struggling. But he was no longer *thriving*, and he knew the difference.

Michael didn't come to me because he'd hit a breaking point. He came because he could see one approaching and wanted to change course before he got there. The difference between reactive and proactive medicine is what separates recovery from longevity.

Every patient in this book so far arrived in crisis. Sarah's gut had collapsed. James's mitochondria were failing. Emma's thyroid was under attack. Alex's neurotransmitters were depleted. Claire's methylation could not support pregnancy. Marcus's detox pathways were genetically bottlenecked. Rachel's building was poisoning her family. Each of them needed the system restored before they could think about the future.

Michael was the first patient in this book who walked in and asked a different question: *What can I do now, while I still have capacity, to extend the years I spend feeling like this?*

That is the longevity question. And it changes everything about how you use this framework.

Healthspan Versus Lifespan

Longevity is not just about living longer. It is about living well for longer — staying sharp, strong, and independent right to the end, rather than spending your final decades in managed deterioration.

The distinction between lifespan and healthspan is the most important concept in modern preventive medicine. Your lifespan is how many years you are alive. Your healthspan is how many of those years you spend fit, capable, mentally sharp, and physically independent. For most people, healthspan ends long before lifespan does.

That is what Michael wanted — to close the gap between the two. And the science now supports the idea that this is measurable, trackable, and modifiable.

Your Body Has Two Ages

Until recently, biological age was an abstraction, a concept without a ruler. That has changed. Steve Horvath's landmark 2013 paper demonstrated that DNA methylation patterns could predict biological age with remarkable accuracy, and, more importantly, that the gap between biological and chronological age was associated with disease risk and mortality. His work opened the field. Epigenetic clocks, tools that measure DNA methylation patterns in blood, can now estimate how old your body is functionally, regardless of how many birthdays you have had. More importantly, newer clocks like DunedinPACE do not just measure your biological age at a single point. They measure the *pace* at which you are ageing, how fast or slow the process is moving. That means you can test, intervene, and retest to see whether the intervention is slowing the biological clock.

Two clocks have emerged as the most clinically useful: GrimAge, which estimates biological age and mortality risk from DNA methylation patterns, and DunedinPACE, which measures the rate of ageing rather than just where the clock currently sits. Both are trackable. Both respond to intervention. These tests are now available worldwide through practitioner-ordered epigenetic testing kits, with new organ-specific and immune-ageing clocks emerging every year. Ask your functional medicine practitioner, or visit thehealinghierarchy.com for current testing options in your region.

The same retesting philosophy this book has applied to gut markers, methylation, hormones, and neurotransmitters now applies to ageing itself. Research published in 2024 confirmed that different organs age at different rates inside the same person. Your heart can be biologically older than your brain, your immune system younger than your liver. Those with biologically older hearts had dramatically higher risk of heart failure. Those whose brain and immune system both tested as biologically young had significantly lower mortality over fifteen years. The body doesn't age uniformly. Each system has its own trajectory, and each can be influenced independently.

This is the systems-thinking this entire book has been teaching, applied to the biology of ageing. You aren't simply "getting older." Specific systems are declining at specific rates for specific, identifiable reasons. Those reasons are largely the same upstream drivers we have been addressing throughout every case: inflammation, oxidative stress, nutrient depletion, mitochondrial decline, and hormonal drift.

Aging Happens in Waves

One of the most important findings in recent ageing research is that biological decline does not follow a smooth, gradual curve. A landmark study tracking molecular changes across the lifespan found that ageing occurs in two dramatic acceleration points. The first wave hits around age forty, when metabolism shifts. The way the body processes fats, caffeine, and alcohol changes measurably, and cardiovascular markers begin to drift. The second wave arrives around age sixty, when immune function weakens significantly, increasing susceptibility to metabolic disease, cognitive decline, and systemic inflammation.

These are not arbitrary numbers. They are windows — transition points where the body's capacity to self-regulate drops and accumulated damage begins to compound. Intervention during these windows has disproportionate impact. Michael arrived at fifty-two — twelve years past the first wave and eight years before the second. He was in the corridor between them, and the data confirmed it.

Michael's Data

Michael's conventional bloods were unremarkable. His GP was right, by standard pathology ranges, nothing was flagged. But standard ranges are designed to detect disease, not to detect drift. The functional investigation told a different story.

Biological age. Estimated at approximately fifty-six — four years older than his chronological age of fifty-two. Michael was ageing faster than the calendar.

Inflammation. CRP was 2.8 mg/L, where optimal is below 1.0. Not high enough to trigger a diagnosis, but high enough to drive vascular ageing, neuroinflammation, and cellular damage over decades. Homocysteine was 10.2 μmol/L, where optimal is below 7. Recent research has established that elevated homocysteine is causally associated with accelerated biological ageing, not only a cardiovascular risk factor. This was the same marker we tracked in Claire's methylation case. In her context, it contributed to pregnancy loss. In Michael's context, it was accelerating the pace at which every system in his body was deteriorating.

Methylation. B12 was 285 pmol/L, technically within range, functionally suboptimal. Folate was low-normal. His methylation cycle was not failing — it was underperforming. Not enough to cause symptoms now. Enough to compound over twenty years.

Mitochondrial function. CoQ10 was 0.38 µmol/L, where optimal is above 0.8. OAT showed elevated oxidative stress markers. His mitochondria, the same organelles that failed catastrophically in James's case, were producing less energy and generating more waste. NAD+, the cellular energy currency that declines with age across virtually every tissue, was inferred to be significantly depleted based on surrogate markers and his age-adjusted profile.

Mineral status. HTMA showed low magnesium, low-normal zinc, low selenium, elevated copper, and detectable levels of mercury, lead, and aluminium — low-level but chronic. Not an acute toxicity. A slow, compounding mineral imbalance eroding enzymatic function across hundreds of biochemical pathways.

Hormones. Total testosterone was 380 ng/dL, where the functional optimal range starts at 450. Free testosterone was low-normal. DHEA was declining. His hormonal profile was not deficient — it was drifting. The same pattern James experienced, but caught earlier, before the crash.

Gut. GI-MAP showed suboptimal microbial diversity. The Firmicutes-to-Bacteroidetes ratio was skewed. Keystone longevity-associated species, Akkermansia muciniphila, Faecalibacterium prausnitzii, were low. His gut was not diseased. It was ageing.

No single marker was alarming, but every marker was drifting in the wrong direction. That is what ageing looks like in data. Not a single failure, but a system-wide loss of margin. And it is precisely the kind of pattern that standard pathology, designed for disease detection, will miss entirely until it becomes disease.

What Ageing Actually Is

Ageing is the accumulation of friction across every biological system simultaneously. That friction has specific, measurable components: chronic low-grade inflammation that damages tissues faster than they can repair. Oxidative stress from mitochondria producing more waste and less energy. Nutrient depletion that starves enzymatic reactions of their cofactors. Hormonal decline that reduces the body's capacity to build, repair, and regulate. The accumulation of senescent cells — damaged cells that stop dividing but refuse to die, pumping out inflammatory signals that accelerate the ageing of everything around them. The steady decline of NAD+, the cofactor that powers cellular energy production, DNA repair, and the sirtuin enzymes that regulate gene expression.

Every upstream intervention in this book — gut repair, methylation support, mitochondrial restoration, hormonal rebalancing, detoxification, environmental remediation — reduces one or more of these friction points. That is why the framework does not change when the question shifts from recovery to longevity. The architecture is identical: test, identify the drivers, intervene in sequence, retest, adjust. The only difference is that in recovery, you are restoring lost function. In longevity, you are protecting existing function and building biological reserve.

The Four-Level Longevity Protocol

Level 1 — foundational longevity stack.

Methylation support with a methylated B-complex, activated B12, and P-5-P.

Mitochondrial support with ubiquinol CoQ10, PQQ, and magnesium glycinate.

NAD+ restoration with NMN.

Mineral repletion, zinc, selenium, molybdenum, to correct the deficits HTMA had identified and support copper balancing and sulfite oxidase function.

Gentle ongoing heavy metal clearance with chlorella, modified citrus pectin, and alpha-lipoic acid.

Gut support with a multi-strain probiotic, another probiotic emphasising Akkermansia, combined with prebiotic fibre and fermented foods.

Omega-3 at therapeutic doses for inflammation.

Daily sun exposure for vitamin D, not supplementation, but deliberate time outdoors, because the body produces vitamin D most effectively through direct UVB exposure on skin, and the downstream benefits of sunlight extend beyond vitamin D alone to include circadian regulation, nitric oxide production, and immune modulation.

Level 2 — advanced longevity compounds.

NMN at 500 to 1,000 mg daily for NAD+ restoration. The cellular energy currency that declines measurably with age and whose depletion is now linked to mitochondrial dysfunction, impaired DNA repair, and accelerated cellular ageing across multiple tissues.

Senolytic compounds, quercetin and fisetin, pulse-dosed rather than taken continuously, because senescent cells accumulate slowly and intermittent clearance is more effective and better tolerated than daily dosing.

Autophagy enhancers including spermidine and resveratrol to support the body's cellular recycling systems.

Longevity polyphenols — EGCG, pterostilbene, to support antioxidant defence and gene expression.

Carnosine for glycation inhibition.

Natural testosterone support through zinc optimisation, ashwagandha (KSM-66), and herbal compounds including Tongkat Ali.

No TRT, because Michael's testosterone decline was upstream-driven, not primary.

Level 3 — lifestyle as medicine. This is where the protocol either works or fails. The supplements provide the biochemical foundation. The lifestyle provides the physiological stimulus.

Exercise structured around three modalities: Zone 2 cardiovascular training four times per week for mitochondrial density and metabolic health, resistance training three times per week to preserve muscle mass, bone density, and insulin sensitivity, because muscle is metabolic currency and sarcopenia is one of the strongest predictors of all-cause mortality, and VO_2 max intervals once per week to maintain cardiovascular capacity.

Nutrition built around a whole-food, anti-inflammatory base with adequate protein at 1.6 to 2.0 grams per kilogram of body weight, rich in polyphenols, with intermittent fasting at 16:8 daily and quarterly three-day fasts to activate autophagy.

Sleep optimised at seven to eight hours with circadian consistency, magnesium glycinate and L-theanine before bed, and blue light eliminated two hours before sleep.

Stress modulation through sauna three to four times per week for heat shock protein activation and cardiovascular benefit, cold exposure two to three times per week for metabolic resilience and immune function — appropriate here because Michael's HPA axis was fully stabilised, his sleep was optimised, and his nervous system had the capacity to recover from the hormetic stress — breathwork, and deliberate investment in purpose and social connection, because the longest-lived populations in the world, from Okinawa to Sardinia to Ikaria, share these traits more consistently than any supplement protocol.

Level 4 — monitoring and iteration. This is what separates longevity practice from longevity theatre. The performance of health-optimising behaviours without the feedback loop that confirms whether they are working.

Every three to six months: inflammatory markers (CRP, homocysteine), metabolic health (fasting glucose, insulin, HbA1c, lipid panel), hormone panel (testosterone, DHEA, thyroid), micronutrient status (vitamin D, B12, folate, magnesium, zinc).

Mitochondrial function (CoQ10, OAT markers annually).

HTMA retested at nine to twelve months to track mineral repletion and heavy metal clearance.

Gut microbiome diversity assessed annually.

Biological age markers, epigenetic clocks including GrimAge and DunedinPACE, tracked to confirm whether the intervention is slowing the biological clock or merely improving surrogate markers.

The protocol is not static — the data drives every adjustment. Longevity is a skill. You get better at it over time.

The Outcome

Twelve months later, Michael's data told a story that standard medicine would never have predicted, because standard medicine would never have tested for it.

Biological age had dropped from approximately fifty-six to approximately forty-eight — an eight-year reversal. At fifty-three, his biology now resembled someone five years younger than his chronological age. CRP had fallen from 2.8 to 0.4, optimal. Homocysteine from 10.2 to 6.1, optimal, and no longer driving accelerated biological ageing. B12 was above 500. Folate was optimal. CoQ10 had risen from 0.38 to 1.1 —

optimal, with OAT oxidative stress markers normalised. Minerals were optimised across the board — magnesium, zinc, selenium all in range, copper normalised, heavy metals significantly reduced. Gut diversity had improved, with keystone longevity species restored and a microbiome profile resembling someone decades younger.

Testosterone had climbed from 380 to 620 ng/dL, without TRT. No hormone replacement. No pharmaceutical intervention. Upstream optimisation alone — zinc repletion, inflammation reduction, sleep improvement, heavy metal clearance, stress modulation, had allowed his endocrine system to recover its own production. The same principle demonstrated in James's case, applied proactively rather than reactively. This isn't universal. Some men require TRT, and there is no failure in that. Michael's decline was upstream-driven, which meant upstream correction was sufficient.

When I asked Michael how he felt twelve months in, he didn't hesitate.

'Honestly? Better than I did at forty-five. My recovery is faster, my focus is sharper, I'm sleeping properly for the first time in years. And I'm not dreading what's coming anymore. I actually feel like I've got a handle on it.'

He smiled. 'The funny thing is, my mates think I'm doing something extreme. I'm not. I'm just following a plan.

Longevity Is a Practice, Not a Protocol

Michael's case is different from every other case in this book in one critical respect: there was no crisis to resolve. No system had failed. No threshold had been crossed. He came with resilience still intact and asked how to protect it. That shift, from reactive to proactive, from "what went wrong" to "how do I stay right", is the transition from recovery to longevity.

None of that changes. Data still drives every decision. Sequence still matters. You can't optimise hormones while inflammation is uncontrolled;

you can't support mitochondria while mineral cofactors are depleted; you can't build biological reserve while the gut is compromised. The architecture is identical, but the intention is different. Recovery is about restoring what was lost. Longevity is about building what will be needed.

Eight cases across eight chapters. Sarah, James, Emma, Alex, Claire, Marcus, Rachel, Michael. Each entered the framework at a different point and with a different driver. Each demonstrated that the same framework, test, sequence, restore, monitor, applies whether the system has collapsed or is simply drifting. The only variable is when you begin.

Most people begin when they have no choice. Michael began when he still had every choice. That is the longevity advantage. Not a supplement. Not a protocol. A decision to treat ageing as something you can influence rather than something that happens to you.

Longevity is not about only living longer. It is about living well for longer. The body doesn't care about your age. It cares about your biology. Change the biology, and the trajectory changes with it. The only question is when you decide to begin.

MICHAEL — Longevity Optimisation (12 months)

MARKER	BEFORE		AFTER
Biological Age	56 years	→	48 years
CRP	2.8 mg/L	→	0.4 mg/L
Testosterone	380 ng/dL	→	620 ng/dL
Fasting Insulin	Elevated	→	Optimised
Homocysteine	Borderline	→	Optimal
Vitamin D	Suboptimal	→	Optimised

Biological age reversed 8 years. Inflammatory markers normalised.

Michael's longevity protocol is available at TheHealingHierarchy.com.

For optimizing complex cases, particularly those involving multi-system hormonal failure, long-standing treatment resistance, or advanced longevity optimisation — one-on-one consultations are available at jarrodcoopernd.com.

PART VIII
THE FRAMEWORK

Chapter Nineteen

The Framework You can Trust

This book has taken you through eight patients, eight drivers, and a single architecture that resolved every one of them. Sarah's gut. James's mitochondria. Emma's thyroid. Alex's neurotransmitters. Claire's methylation. Marcus's detox pathways. Rachel's environment. Michael's biological age. Each case was different. Each investigation led somewhere distinct. But the framework that guided every decision was identical.

Test. Sequence. Restore. Monitor. Adjust.

That sequence is not a protocol. It is a way of thinking about recovery. Protocols expire. Protocols belong to the moment they were designed for. The specific combination of symptoms, lab values, and physiological load that existed when they were written. The moment any one of those variables changes, the protocol becomes incomplete. That is why protocols fail over time and why patients who follow them perfectly still plateau, regress, or feel lost when their initial gains stall.

This approach does not expire. It adapts. It asks the same questions no matter what the body is doing: What is the data showing? What is the upstream driver? What is the correct sequence of intervention? Is the intervention working? If not, what has changed? Those questions are as useful on day one of a health crisis as they are ten years into a longevity practice. This chapter is about making that framework yours, not as a reader following instructions, but as someone who understands the logic well enough to apply it independently for the rest of your life.

The Operating System

Every case in this book followed the same decision architecture, whether the patient was in crisis or optimising. That framework has four layers.

1. **Foundations first.** Foundations first — but not foundations alone. When a client begins, we start testing immediately and begin targeted supplementation as soon as the data comes back. But that supplementation works best when the fundamentals are running alongside it. Diet. Sleep. Movement. Nervous system regulation. Hydration. Blood sugar stability. These comprise the non-negotiable platform upon which every intervention depends, regardless of how advanced the case. Sarah's gut protocol wouldn't have worked without the dietary changes that accompanied it. James's mitochondrial support would not have restored his energy if his sleep architecture had remained fragmented. Alex's neurotransmitter recovery was built on a nervous system that had first been stabilised. The foundations aren't a phase you complete before treatment begins. They're the operating system that makes treatment work. Skip them, and everything you build on top will be unstable

2. **Data to clarify.** The Essential Trilogy, comprehensive stool test, organic acids test, and functional blood panel, provides a three-dimensional map of what is happening inside the body. Not what a single blood test suggests might be happening. Not what symptoms imply. Not what the internet has convinced you is wrong. Data removes guesswork. Data reveals drivers that symptoms alone cannot distinguish. Emma's thyroid antibodies were invisible on a standard thyroid panel. Claire's active B12 told a completely different story from her serum B12. Marcus's stool test was largely unremarkable while his organic acids test revealed catastrophic detox failure. No single test tells the whole story.

The trilogy exists because the body is a system, and systems require triangulation.

3. **Sequence to prioritise.** Knowing what is wrong is not enough. You must know what to fix first. The healing hierarchy is the order of operations that determines whether an intervention succeeds or fails. Gut before hormones, because you can't absorb the nutrients required to build hormones through a damaged intestinal barrier. Inflammation before optimisation, because an immune system in overdrive will override every supplement you add. Detox capacity before detox protocols, because mobilising toxins without the enzymatic machinery to process them produces redistribution, not clearance. Methylation support before hormonal optimisation, because the enzymes that metabolise hormones depend on methylation pathways. Every practitioner in this book who had treated these patients before me was not wrong about what was broken. They were wrong about the order in which it should be repaired. Sequence is not a detail. Sequence is the strategy.

4. **Adjustment based on impact.** The protocol you start with is never the protocol you finish with. Every intervention changes the internal environment, which changes what the body needs next. Retesting various markers at three, six, and twelve months is the mechanism by which the framework stays accurate. Sarah's gut protocol shifted at month six when her retest showed the infection had cleared but her zonulin was still elevated. Emma's thyroid support was adjusted when her antibodies dropped but her T3 conversion remained sluggish. Michael's longevity stack will evolve every year as his biological age markers and metabolic profile change. Adjustment is not failure. Adjustment is the strategy. A framework that doesn't adjust is a protocol pretending to be a framework.

Why Protocol Hopping Fails

Most patients who come to me have already tried multiple approaches. They have done elimination diets, gut cleanses, hormone protocols, methylation support, detox programs, and supplement stacks recommended by practitioners, podcasts, or online communities. Some of these interventions helped temporarily. Most stopped working. And the patient concluded either that functional medicine does not work or that their body is uniquely broken.

Neither conclusion is correct. What happened is protocol hopping, moving from one intervention to the next without a method to determine whether the intervention was appropriate, whether it was given enough time, whether it was sequenced correctly, or whether it actually worked. Protocol hopping is the natural consequence of treating symptoms without understanding systems. When the symptom improves, the patient assumes the protocol worked. When the symptom returns, the patient assumes the protocol stopped working and moves to the next one. But the symptom was never the target. The upstream driver was. Unless the upstream driver was identified and resolved, the symptom was always going to return, regardless of which protocol temporarily suppressed it.

The antidote to protocol hopping is not a better protocol. It is a better question. Instead of asking: *What should I take for this symptom?* the framework asks: *What upstream system is feeding this symptom, and has it been addressed in the correct sequence?* That question, applied reliably, eliminates most of the confusion that drives patients from practitioner to practitioner and protocol to protocol.

How to Use This Framework For Yourself

Give interventions time: the gut takes three to six months to repair, mitochondrial function takes four to eight months to restore, Hormonal rebalancing takes six to twelve months. Methylation pathways do not normalise in just weeks. Heavy metals do not clear in a single round of chelation. Biological age does not reverse in ninety days. If you change protocols every four to six weeks based on how you feel, you will never know whether any of them were working. The minimum assessment window for any meaningful intervention is three months. For complex or multi-system cases, six months. If you retest at that point and the data has not moved, then you change course, because the data told you to, not because your anxiety did.

Retest to confirm. Symptoms are feedback, but they are unreliable narrators. A patient can feel better while their inflammatory markers are still elevated. A patient can feel worse during a Herxheimer reaction while their gut markers are improving. A patient can feel no different while their methylation markers are normalising. Feeling better is not proof of healing. Feeling worse is not proof of failure. The data confirms what is happening beneath the symptom surface. Retesting is not an expense. It is the only reliable way to know whether to continue, adjust, or change direction entirely.

Adjust based on data, not anxiety. The urge to change course when progress stalls is natural. It is also almost always premature. Healing is not linear — there are plateaus where nothing appears to be changing. There are flares where symptoms temporarily worsen as the body recalibrates. There are periods where one system improves while another appears to regress, because restoring one pathway increases demand on another. These are normal features of multi-system recovery, and they look exactly like failure unless you have the data to show they aren't. The framework protects you from your own impatience. Trust the data. Adjust when the data says to adjust. Not before.

Healing Is Not Linear

This is the single most important expectation to set, and the one most commonly violated. Healing does not follow a straight upward line. It follows a trajectory that includes setbacks, plateaus, flares, and periods of apparent stagnation that are, in fact, the body reorganising at a deeper level.

Die-off reactions — Herxheimer responses — happen when pathogens are cleared faster than the body can process the debris. They feel like regression. They are evidence that the intervention is working.

Hormonal recalibration produces mood swings, sleep changes, and energy fluctuations before it produces stability.

Gut repair involves periods where digestion temporarily worsens as the microbiome shifts. Detoxification mobilises stored toxins that can cause headaches, fatigue, and brain fog before they are eliminated.

Every one of these is a predictable phase of recovery, not a sign that something has gone wrong.

The patients who recover most completely are not the ones who never experience setbacks. They are the ones who understand that setbacks are part of the process and who have the data to distinguish a temporary recalibration from a genuine regression requiring a change in approach. Knowing whether you are looking at a healing crisis or a treatment failure is one of the most important clinical judgments in functional medicine. It is one that a framework-driven approach handles far better than a symptom-driven one, because the framework asks: *What does the data say?* not *How does the patient feel today?*

Adjustment Is Permanent

There is no point at which you are "done." This is a way of interacting with your own biology for the rest of your life, not a twelve-week program. The variables that affect your health — stress, sleep quality, dietary changes, environmental exposures, hormonal shifts, ageing itself - are not static. They change continuously. Which means the body's needs change continuously. Which means the interventions that support those needs must change continuously.

Sarah recovered from gut dysfunction and felt well for three years before a period of sustained work stress caused her zonulin to climb and her symptoms to return. That was a new load on a system that had been stable but not invulnerable. The framework told her exactly what to do: retest, identify the driver, intervene. She needed a targeted adjustment to a system she already understood. Within ten weeks of the adjusted protocol, her symptoms had resolved again. The framework had not failed her the first time. Life had loaded the system. The framework simply told her what to do about it.

Michael's longevity protocol will look different at sixty than it does at fifty-three. His hormonal needs will shift. His mitochondrial demands will increase. His methylation requirements may change with new genetic expression patterns that emerge with age. The protocol he is on today is not the protocol he will be on in five years. But the framework that determines what protocol he should be on will be exactly the same.

That is the difference between a protocol and a way of thinking. A protocol gives you a plan. A framework gives you the ability to make your own plans — forever.

Thinking Like a Clinical Engineer

The preceding sections tell you what to do. This section tells you how to think, so that you can determine the right steps independently of any practitioner, protocol, or supplement list. Throughout this book, the approach to every patient has followed the same logic: trace the symptom upstream to its driver, identify which system is failing and why, determine the correct sequence of repair, intervene, retest, and adjust. That is clinical engineering. The systematic diagnosis and repair of biological systems using data, sequence, and iteration.

You can apply this same logic to yourself. When a symptom appears, do not ask: *What should I take for this?* Ask: *What upstream system is feeding this?* When an intervention stops working, do not assume it has failed. Ask: *What has changed? What is the new bottleneck?* When you feel stuck, do not just add more supplements. Ask: *Have I retested? Do I actually know what the data says right now?* When progress stalls, do not change everything at once. Ask: *Is this a plateau, a healing crisis, or a genuine regression.? Which one does the data support?*

Think in systems, not symptoms. Think in sequences, not silver bullets. Think in trajectories, not snapshots. A single lab value at a single point in time tells you almost nothing. A series of lab values over six to twelve months tells you almost everything. The body is a system to be understood continuously, not a puzzle to be solved once. The body is not unpredictable. It is usually unmeasured.

What the Framework Gives You

At the beginning of this book, most readers were stuck. Stuck in a cycle of symptoms, specialists, and supplements that produced temporary relief but no lasting resolution. Stuck wondering whether their body was fundamentally broken or whether they simply hadn't found the right practitioner yet. Stuck oscillating between hope and resignation with every new protocol and every new setback.

This approach does not promise that you will never be unwell again. It promises something more useful: that you will never be confused about what to do next. When symptoms appear, you have a method. When interventions stall, you have a diagnostic logic. When life changes, new stress, new environment, new phase of ageing, you have a framework that adapts with you.

You are no longer dependent on a practitioner to tell you what is wrong. You are no longer dependent on a protocol to tell you what to take. You are no longer guessing. You understand how your body works as a system. You understand how to test it, how to read the results, how to intervene in the correct order, and how to confirm whether the intervention is working. That is literacy, and it stays with you.

The Practice, Not the Destination

Healing is not a destination. It is a practice, and one that deepens over time as your understanding of your own biology sharpens. The first time you read your blood panel with functional ranges rather than pathology ranges, you see things your GP never mentioned. The first time you correlate your stool test with your organic acids test, you understand why a gut protocol alone was never going to resolve your symptoms. The first time you retest and see the numbers move in the direction you predicted, you stop feeling like a passive patient and start feeling like someone who understands their own biology.

That shift, from passenger to navigator, is the real outcome of this book. Not any single supplement. Not any single case study. Not any single lab value. The ability to think about your health the way an engineer thinks about a system: with curiosity, with data, with sequence, and with the patience to let the process unfold.

There will always be new challenges. New stressors. New phases of life that change what your body needs. But you now have a system that handles all of them. Not because it gives you all the answers in advance, but because it gives you the method to find the right answer every time.

The testing resources, supplement protocols, and clinical tools referenced throughout this book are available at TheHealingHierarchy.com. This is a living resource — updated as the evidence evolves and as the framework is refined through clinical practice.

> *You aren't broken. You never were. You were unmeasured. Now you have the framework to measure, the sequence to act, and the data to know whether it is working.*

Conclusion

There is a version of your life on the other side of this work that you may not be able to imagine yet.

You wake up and your energy is already there. Not borrowed from caffeine. Not conditional on a perfect night's sleep. Just present. The way it used to be before you stopped trusting it. Your thinking is clear. Not the foggy, effortful concentration you have learned to push through, but genuine clarity, the kind where ideas arrive cleanly and decisions feel clear. Your digestion works without negotiation. Your mood is stable without being managed. You eat without fear. You exercise and recover. You handle stress and come back to baseline. You sleep and wake feeling like sleep did something.

That is not an aspirational fantasy. It is what the body is capable of when you stop guessing and start reading the map it has been giving you all along. Sarah said it felt like someone had turned the volume down on everything that had been screaming at her for years. James said he didn't realise how much energy he had been spending just coping until he no longer had to. Emma said the strangest part was realising she had forgotten what better felt like. Alex said the anxiety did not lift all at once; one day he simply noticed it was no longer the first thing he felt when he opened his eyes.

These are what the body does when you stop fighting it and start understanding it. Claire, Marcus, Rachel, and Michael said versions of the same thing, in their own language. The words were different. The pattern was identical.

What You Now Understand

You came to this book because something was not working. Perhaps you had been unwell for a long time and conventional medicine had not found a cause. Perhaps you had been given a diagnosis but the treatment had not resolved the symptoms. Perhaps you had done everything you were told, eaten well, exercised, managed your stress, taken the supplements, and still felt like your body was working against you.

You now understand why.

Your body wasn't failing randomly. It had crossed a threshold. A point where the accumulated load on your biological systems exceeded what the body could handle. Once that threshold was crossed, the same inputs that had kept you well before stopped working. Food that had been fine started producing symptoms. Sleep that had been restorative stopped restoring. Exercise that had built you up started breaking you down. The problem was never effort. The problem was never willpower. The problem was a system operating beyond its capacity to regulate, and no amount of good intention can fix a regulatory failure.

What fixes it is what this book has laid out across nineteen chapters: identify the upstream driver, restore the system in the correct sequence, and use data, not symptoms, to confirm that the intervention is working.

Clarity came first. You stopped guessing. You learned to see the body as an interconnected system rather than a collection of isolated symptoms, and you learned that those systems fail in sequence and recover in sequence.

Recovery came next. Not through more effort, but through a better framework. Removing what was stealing your body's ability to heal, mattered more than adding another supplement to an already overwhelmed system.

Resilience followed. Not the motivational poster kind, the biological kind. The gap between where your body sits today and the point where it starts to break down. The goal was never just to feel better. It was to build enough buffer that feeling better actually lasts.

Three Things Worth Remembering

If you take nothing else from this book, take these points.

Most people do not fall apart all at once. There is a moment, one stressor too many, one system too depleted, when the body stops coping the way it used to. That moment is when the body crosses its threshold. Recognising it is where real recovery begins.

Your symptoms were never random. They were the result of a system operating beyond what it could regulate. Every symptom had an upstream driver. Every driver had a sequence in which it needed to be addressed. The architecture of recovery is precise.

The body was never the enemy. It was responding to conditions. Change the conditions, in the right order, confirmed by data, and the outcome changes with them.

Where to Go From Here

You have finished the book. What matters now is what you do with it.

Start with the free Implementation Workbook at TheHealingHierarchy.com/workbook. It turns the framework into something personal. Then score yourself one more time using the Stability Score from Chapter 2. That number will tell you where to begin, and the next section will show you exactly what each score means for your path forward.

There is no rush. The door is open when you are ready.

The Map Is Yours

Sarah arrived after her system had already crossed the threshold. She had been unwell long enough to doubt whether recovery was still possible. She recovered and now understands how to maintain what she rebuilt. Michael did not wait for the crossing. He recognised the narrowing margin early and acted before the threshold compounded. Both recovered, both now hold the same framework. The difference was timing.

You have that same choice now.

You came to the end of this book the same way you came to the beginning — looking for answers. The difference is that you now know where to look. You know what to test. You know what sequence to follow. You know what questions to ask. And you know that the body is not unpredictable. It is unmeasured until you decide to measure it.

Your body didn't fail you.

It crossed a threshold.

And now you know how to cross back.

Your Free Implementation Workbook

This book gave you the framework. The workbook makes it personal.

The companion Implementation Workbook follows the book chapter by chapter — 19 exercises that turn what you read into what you do. Each one takes ten to fifteen minutes. It is free and it is yours.

Readers consistently tell me this is the moment the book stops being theory and starts being theirs.

Download it free at TheHealingHierarchy.com/workbook

One Sentence Could Change Someone's Health

If this book changed how you understand your health, even one concept, one chapter, one shift in how you see what your body has been doing, I have a small request.

Leave a short review on the platform where you purchased it.

Not for me. For the person who is still searching. The one cycling through supplements that aren't working, seeing practitioners who cannot find anything wrong, lying awake wondering if this is just who they are now. That person is one book away from understanding why their body stopped responding, and your review may be the reason they pick this one up instead of another protocol that sends them further down the wrong path.

You don't need to write a summary. A sentence about what shifted for you is enough. That sentence could be the thing that helps someone finally stop searching in the wrong places and start recovering.

Thank you for your time with these pages. I don't take it lightly.

Jarrod Cooper - ND

Please leave an Amazon review at TheHealingHierarchy.com/Review

Your Next Step

Before you close this book, score yourself one more time. The same zero-to-ten Stability Score from Chapter 2.

That number tells you where to start.

YOUR PATH FORWARD
YOUR STABILITY SCORE
0 - 3
CRISIS
Clinical Support
jarrodcoopernd.com
4 - 6
FRAGILE
Guided Program
functionalmedicinesolution.com
7+
STABLE
Data & Tools
TheHealingHierarchy.com
Not ready yet? Start with the free workbook
TheHealingHierarchy.com/workbook

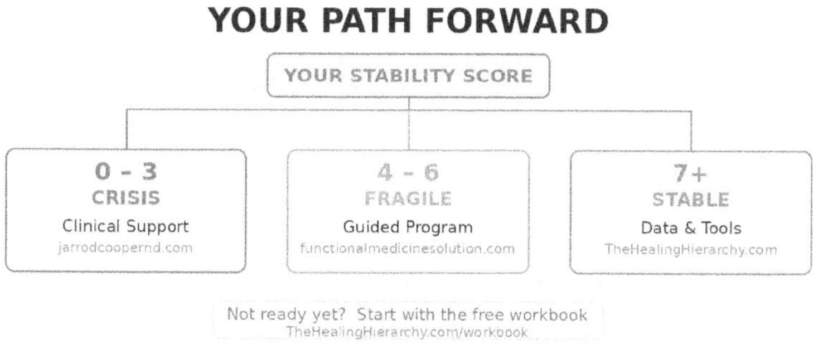

If your score is 0 to 3 — you are in crisis.

Your symptoms are unpredictable. Your life is organised around the illness. Good days are rare and unreliable. You have likely seen multiple practitioners without lasting improvement.

Your case almost certainly has layered complexity — overlapping drivers that need to be identified in sequence and addressed in the right order. The Essential Trilogy testing is the starting point, but the interpretation and clinical strategy around that data benefit from direct support.

Clinical consultations are available for complex cases, particularly those involving CIRS, multi-system autoimmunity, treatment-resistant fatigue, or long-standing hormonal and neurological dysfunction.

If your score is 4 to 6 — you are fragile but improving.

Good days are appearing. But setbacks still happen, and you aren't yet confident the gains will hold. You understand the framework. You may have already started adjusting your foundations. What you need now is structure and clinical oversight to move through the restoration sequence without guesswork.

The Functional Medicine Solution online program translates this framework into guided implementation — step by step, with the same architecture described in this book applied in real time. It includes testing options, interpretation, protocol design, and ongoing support through each phase of the Healing Hierarchy.

If your score is 7 or above — you are stable and building.

Your foundations are solid. Your symptoms are manageable or resolving. You are looking to optimise, track, and stay ahead of any drift rather than recover from crisis. You may not need clinical oversight — you need data and the tools to interpret it.

You can order your Essential Trilogy testing at TheHealingHierarchy.com, stool testing, organic acids, and a functional blood panel, along with the interpretation framework, optimal ranges, supplement protocols, and tracking tools referenced throughout this book.

Whatever your score, your next step starts at TheHealingHierarchy.com. You will find testing, programs, clinical support, and the workbook, each matched to where you are right now.

TheHealingHierarchy.com

If you aren't ready for any of these yet — that is fine. Start with the workbook and stabilise the basics: sleep, nutrition, movement, consistency over perfection. Review any testing you already have through the lens of what you now understand. You may find answers that were already present, waiting for the right framework to make them visible.

The cost of getting the sequence wrong — months of wasted supplements, regression from premature interventions, another year of confusion, is almost always greater than the cost of getting it right the first time. There is no rush. The door is open when you are ready.

Selected References & Further Reading

The following references support the key claims, statistics, and clinical frameworks cited throughout this book. This isn't an exhaustive bibliography but a curated list of the foundational research behind the principles discussed. Readers who wish to explore the science in greater depth will find these papers and texts an excellent starting point.

Chapter 2 — Why Your Body Stopped Responding

McEwen, B.S., & Stellar, E. (1993). Stress and the individual: Mechanisms leading to disease. *Archives of Internal Medicine*, 153(18), 2093–2101.

McEwen, B.S. (1998). Stress, adaptation, and disease: Allostasis and allostatic overload. *Annals of the New York Academy of Sciences*, 840(1), 33–44.

McEwen, B.S. (2008). Central effects of stress hormones in health and disease: Understanding the protective and damaging effects of stress and stress mediators. *European Journal of Pharmacology*, 583(2–3), 174–185.

Chapter 5 — Sleep Is Not a Lifestyle Problem

Walker, M. (2017). *Why We Sleep: Unlocking the Power of Sleep and Dreams*. Scribner.

Irwin, M.R. (2015). Why sleep is important for health: A psychoneuroimmunology perspective. *Annual Review of Psychology*, 66, 143–172.

Chapter 7 — The Nervous System Is Not a Mindset Problem

Porges, S.W. (2011). *The Polyvagal Theory: Neurophysiological Foundations of Emotions, Attachment, Communication, and Self-Regulation*. W.W. Norton.

Breit, S., Kupferberg, A., Rogler, G., & Hasler, G. (2018). Vagus nerve as modulator of the brain–gut axis in psychiatric and inflammatory disorders. *Frontiers in Psychiatry*, 9, 44.

Beecher, H.K. (1955). The powerful placebo. *Journal of the American Medical Association*, 159(17), 1602–1606. [Origin of the widely cited finding that placebo responses account for approximately 35% of therapeutic effect in clinical trials.]

Hróbjartsson, A., & Gøtzsche, P.C. (2001). Is the placebo powerless? An analysis of clinical trials comparing placebo with no treatment. *New England Journal of Medicine*, 344(21), 1594–1602. [Systematic review testing and refining the placebo response literature.]

Chapter 10 — The Gut: Health Begins Here

Vighi, G., Marcucci, F., Sensi, L., Di Cara, G., & Frati, F. (2008). Allergy and the gastrointestinal system. *Clinical & Experimental Immunology*, 153(S1), 3–16. [70–80% of immune system housed in gut-associated lymphoid tissue.]

Yano, J.M., Yu, K., Donaldson, G.P., et al. (2015). Indigenous bacteria from the gut microbiota regulate host serotonin biosynthesis. *Cell*, 161(2), 264–276. [Approximately 95% of serotonin produced in the gastrointestinal tract.]

Cryan, J.F., & Dinan, T.G. (2012). Mind-altering microorganisms: The impact of the gut microbiota on brain and behaviour. *Nature Reviews Neuroscience*, 13(10), 701–712.

Chapter 12 — Hormones Are Downstream

Fasano, A. (2011). Zonulin and its regulation of intestinal barrier function: The biological door to inflammation, autoimmunity, and cancer. *Physiological Reviews*, 91(1), 151–175.

Fasano, A. (2012). Leaky gut and autoimmune diseases. *Clinical Reviews in Allergy & Immunology*, 42(1), 71–78.

Vojdani, A., Kharrazian, D., & Mukherjee, P.S. (2014). The prevalence of antibodies against wheat and milk proteins in blood donors and their contribution to neuroimmune reactivities. *Nutrients*, 6(1), 15–36. [Molecular mimicry — gluten and thyroid tissue.]

Fournier, A., Berrino, F., Riboli, E., Avenel, V., & Clavel-Chapelon, F. (2005). Breast cancer risk in relation to different types of hormone replacement therapy in the E3N-EPIC cohort. *International Journal of Cancer*, 114(3), 448–454. [Estrogen combined with micronized progesterone showed no increased breast cancer risk (RR 0.9), versus synthetic progestins (RR 1.4).]

Fournier, A., Berrino, F., & Clavel-Chapelon, F. (2008). Unequal risks for breast cancer associated with different hormone replacement therapies: Results from the E3N cohort study. *Breast Cancer Research and Treatment*, 107(1), 103–111. [80,377 women, up to 12 years follow-up. Estrogen-progesterone RR 1.00; estrogen-other progestagens RR 1.69.]

Holtorf, K. (2009). The bioidentical hormone debate: Are bioidentical hormones (estradiol, estriol, and progesterone) safer or more efficacious than commonly used synthetic versions in hormone replacement therapy? *Postgraduate Medicine*, 121(1), 73–85.

Chapter 13 — What Looks Like a Mind Problem Is Usually a Brain Problem

Walsh, W.J. (2012). *Nutrient Power: Heal Your Biochemistry and Heal Your Brain*. Skyhorse Publishing.

Chapter 15 — When Genetics Meet Depletion

Lynch, B. (2018). *Dirty Genes: A Breakthrough Program to Treat the Root Cause of Illness and Optimize Your Health*. HarperOne.

Liew, S.C., & Gupta, E.D. (2015). Methylenetetrahydrofolate reductase (MTHFR) C677T polymorphism: Epidemiology, metabolism and the associated diseases. *European Journal of Medical Genetics*, 58(1), 1–10. [Approximately 40% of the population carries at least one MTHFR variant.]

Negro, R., Schwartz, A., Gismondi, R., Tinelli, A., Mangieri, T., & Stagnaro-Green, A. (2010). Increased pregnancy loss rate in thyroid antibody negative women with TSH levels between 2.5 and 5.0 in the first trimester of pregnancy. *Journal of Clinical Endocrinology & Metabolism*, 95(9), E44–E48. [Higher TSH in early pregnancy associated with increased miscarriage risk.]

Benhadi, N., Wiersinga, W.M., Reitsma, J.B., Vrijkotte, T.G., & Bonsel, G.J. (2009). Higher maternal TSH levels in pregnancy are associated with increased risk for miscarriage, fetal or neonatal death. *European Journal of Endocrinology*, 160(6), 985–991.

Thangaratinam, S., Tan, A., Knox, E., Kilby, M.D., Franklyn, J., & Coomarasamy, A. (2011). Association between thyroid autoantibodies and miscarriage and preterm birth: Meta-analysis of evidence. *BMJ*, 342, d2616.

Chapter 17 — When the Building Is the Problem

Shoemaker, R.C. (2010). *Surviving Mold: Life in the Era of Dangerous Buildings*. Otter Bay Books.

Brewer, J.H., Thrasher, J.D., Straus, D.C., Madison, R.A., & Hooper, D. (2013). Detection of mycotoxins in patients with chronic fatigue syndrome. *Toxins*, 5(4), 605–617.

Shoemaker, R.C., & House, D.E. (2006). Sick building syndrome (SBS) and exposure to water-damaged buildings: Time series study, clinical trial, and mechanisms. *Neurotoxicology and Teratology*, 28(5), 573–588. [Approximately 24% of the population carries HLA gene variants conferring biotoxin susceptibility.]

Chapter 18 — The Longevity Question

Horvath, S. (2013). DNA methylation age of human tissues and cell types. *Genome Biology*, 14(10), R115.

Belsky, D.W., Caspi, A., Corcoran, D.L., et al. (2022). DunedinPACE, a DNA methylation biomarker of the pace of aging. *eLife*, 11, e73420.

Oh, H.S.H., Rutledge, J., Nachun, D., et al. (2023). Organ aging signatures in the plasma proteome track health and disease. *Nature*, 624(7990), 164–172. [Different organs age at different rates within the same individual.]

Shen, X., Wang, C., Zhou, X., et al. (2024). Nonlinear dynamics of multi-omics profiles during human aging. *Nature Aging*, 4, 1619–1634. [Two dramatic waves of biological ageing — around age 40 and age 60.]

About the author

Jarrod Cooper is a naturopathic doctor and one of Australia's leading functional medicine practitioners, known for his work with complex, treatment-resistant chronic illness. Based in Perth, Western Australia, he consults with patients across Australia and worldwide via telehealth.

His practice draws the cases other practitioners cannot solve — patients who have seen multiple specialists, run extensive testing, and followed every recommended protocol without lasting improvement. Most arrive having already exhausted both conventional and functional approaches. The framework in this book was built from those cases.

Over more than a decade of clinical practice and thousands of complex cases, Jarrod has pioneered a sequenced, data-driven approach to multi-system restoration — identifying upstream drivers through advanced functional testing and addressing them in the order the body can respond to, rather than treating the loudest symptom first. His methodology integrates epigenetics, methylation science, clinical biochemistry, and gut-immune modelling into a single decision-making architecture.

He holds a Bachelor of Health Science (Naturopathy), is a Fellow Member of the Australian Natural Therapies Association (ANTA), and a member of the Institute of Functional Medicine (IFM). He is the founder of Advanced Functional Medicine and the creator of the Functional Medicine Solution program.

When he is not in clinic or writing, he is with his partner Gemma and their six children. He lives in Perth, Western Australia.

Connect: TheHealingHierarchy.com

The Program: functionalmedicinesolution.com

Clinical Consultations: jarrodcoopernd.com

Follow: @jarrodcoopernd

www.ingramcontent.com/pod-product-compliance
Lightning Source LLC
LaVergne TN
LVHW010609100826
845148LV00014B/2897

9781764571104